ESSENTIALS
of
TIBETAN
TRADITIONAL
MEDICINE

ESSENTIALS
of
TIBETAN
TRADITIONAL
MEDICINE

AMCHI Thinley Gyatso
and
Chris Hakim DTCM

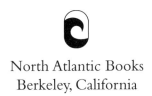

North Atlantic Books
Berkeley, California

Published by
North Atlantic Books
Berkeley, California

Cover art from *Tibetan Medical Paintings* (Serindia Press)
Cover and book design by Susan Quasha
Printed in the United States of America

Essentials of Tibetan Traditional Medicine is sponsored and published by the Society for the Study of Native Arts and Sciences (dba North Atlantic Books), an educational nonprofit based in Berkeley, California, that collaborates with partners to develop cross-cultural perspectives, nurture holistic views of art, science, the humanities, and healing, and seed personal and global transformation by publishing work on the relationship of body, spirit, and nature.

North Atlantic Books' publications are available through most bookstores. For further information, visit our website at www.northatlanticbooks.com or call 800-733-3000.

Library of Congress Cataloging-in-Publication Data
Gyatso, Thinley.
  Essentials of Tibetan traditional medicine / Thinley Gyatso and Chris Hakim.
     p. ; cm.
  Includes bibliographical references and index.
  ISBN 978-1-55643-867-7
  1. Medicine, Tibetan. I. Hakim, Chris. II. Title.
  [DNLM: 1. Medicine, Tibetan Traditional—methods. 2. Plants, Medicinal. WB 55.T5 G996e 2009]
  R603.T5G93 2009
  610—dc22
                           2009034594

2 3 4 5 6 7 8 9 SHERIDAN 21 20 19 18 17 16

Printed on recycled paper

In the degenerate age, common medicines will be out
of reach for poor people, but there will always be herbs.
And if doctors apply themselves with great compassion,
patients will surely be cured.

— ADAPTED FROM THE *Fourth Tantra of Tibetan medicine*

This book is dedicated to the memory
of the great teachers and doctors
of all the ancient medical traditions.
May we live up to their ideals.

CONTENTS

INTRODUCTION

For many years I have been intrigued by Tibetan medicine. In 1989, having just begun the study of traditional Chinese medicine, I attended a Medicine Buddha empowerment with the late Dr. Trogawa Rinpoche. This event was followed by a series of lectures, during which he described various aspects of Tibetan medicine, including the preparation of jewel pills, in some detail, offering a glimpse of a tradition largely unknown in the West. Over time I became fascinated with accounts of accurate diagnoses given simply by examining a patient's pulse, and occasional mention of people being cured of cancer by seemingly simple herbal remedies. But while the study of Chinese medicine was easily available, Tibetan medicine remained mysterious, if only because of the lack of literature in English and the scarcity of practitioners. At the time I did not think that I would have the opportunity to study Tibetan medicine any further.

In 2002, by then a graduate of traditional Chinese medicine, I felt inspired again and embarked on the study of Tibetan medicine to the extent that I could. In the intervening time many books had appeared, describing various aspects of Tibetan diagnostics, therapeutics, plants and herbal formulas, and so on that made the subject much more accessible. At the time I had made a practice of acquiring most of those books as I became aware of them. I took an in-depth correspondence course offered by the Shang Shung Institute in Conway, Massachusetts. By then a fair amount of material had been published on a variety of topics, mostly at an introductory level and without an aim to train practitioners in a systematic way, except for the correspondence course. I felt a need for a book that would concentrate essential aspects of Tibetan medicine beyond the introductory level, with the aim of readying an aspiring student for the next stage: i.e. some form of clinical apprenticeship, as can sometimes be arranged.

In 2005 I had the good fortune of meeting *amchi* Thinley Gyatso, who graciously accepted to be my tutor. Thinley Gyatso was born in Orissa, India, to a family of humble means but rich in the Vajrayana Buddhist and Tibetan medical traditions. His maternal grandfather was a *dzogchen* practitioner and an herbalist who was especially successful in the treatment of mental disorders. On graduating from high school, Thinley Gyatso was admitted both to an engineering college and to *sman rtsis khang* (pronounced "men tsee kang"), the Tibetan medical college of the Tibetan government in exile. Seeing the opportunity both to serve his community and to keep an ancient tradition alive for the benefit of future generations, without hesitation he chose traditional medicine. For the next five years he studied untiringly, taking no more than six hours of sleep each day, and kept a high academic ranking throughout. In that period of time, he had the opportunity to study with *amchi* Dawa,[1] *amchi* Tenpa Chöpel, *amchi* Tenzin Dakpa,[2] *amchi* Tsering Thakchöd, *amchi* Ngawang Dechen, *amchi* Kyenrup Gyatso, and especially *amchi* Lobsang Chöpel and *amchi* "Gyalpo" Palchog, who had studied at the historical Chagpori medical college in Tibet before its destruction by the Chinese. This private study gave him many opportunities to supplement his medical curriculum with invaluable practical advice on diagnosis, bloodletting, moxibustion, pharmacy, bedside manner, etc. When asked about his experience producing this book, Thinley Gyatso cited the classic analogy of the moon and its reflections in bodies of water. The moon represents the historical Buddha Shakyamuni manifesting as the Medicine Buddha and expounding the principles of medicine. The many bodies of water in which the moon can be seen reflected represent the many beings who receive his teaching, each according to his or her own capacity and propensity, and thus embody various medical cultural traditions. Thus, while acknowledging his own fallibility, Thinley Gyatso hopes to be as true as possible to the Buddha's intent in working to preserve and further the tradition of Tibetan medicine.

My Tibetan remains rudimentary at the time of this writing, but Thinley Gyatso is quite fluent in English and, of course, in his native Tibetan. Over the next several years we met at his house for a few hours at a time, elucidating the meaning of the Four Tantras—that venerable canon of Tibetan medicine—and other sources. This process was at times excruciatingly slow and laborious, for there were a surprising number of ambiguities and nuances that needed to be clarified, often by referring to other texts or by drawing on Thinley Gyatso's experience. Tibetan medical texts, like other Tibetan books, are notorious for being extremely dense and context dependent. Even someone perfectly familiar with the language still needs to understand the unstated meaning. An example taken from Tibetan Buddhist literature is the ubiquitous mention of "mother sentient beings."[3] While there is no question that those three words can be translated accurately, a reader not familiar with the expression will be left puzzled. Properly, Tibetan texts should be seen as support for an oral tradition. A translator intent on conveying the meaning of the phrase will have to add a footnote or some other additional wording. In the case of a

---

[1.] Cited in the bibliography.

[2.] Cited in the bibliography.

[3.] "A traditional phrase expressive of the Mahayana view that all sentient beings at one time or another [because of the fathomless cycle of death and rebirth] have been our mothers and thus should be treated with the utmost love and respect" (Chögyam Trungpa 1993).

medical text, it is likewise not sufficient to translate the words if the context is not likely available to the intended reader. But it is also possible to clutter a translation with an abundance of footnotes and other references, ensuring completeness and accuracy but hindering clarity and usability. As a compromise, it was decided from the outset that the main goal of this work would not be scholarly translation but medical insight. This should be considered a commentary of sorts—that is to say, an earnest attempt at elucidation that does not necessarily have the full value of a trusted source. The authoritative source is the original Tibetan version of the Four Tantras, which is considered an extremely reliable text, and to which the reader is referred for further reflection and study. I apologize in advance for any errors or distortions.

In the first part of this book, foundations covered elsewhere are reviewed in summary form. The reader is assumed to have assimilated this material in greater breadth and depth than is presented here. This information is mostly given in the first two Tantras and readily available in English (Clark 1995; Tenzing Dakpa 2007; Yeshi Donden 1986).

The second part is titled "The Humors" and presents a new translation of essential chapters of the Oral Instruction (Third) Tantra. This is where the humors wind, bile, and phlegm are described in great detail in terms of illnesses, diagnostic methods, and basic treatment approaches. Subsequent chapters describe various aspects of heat, cold, and other fundamental topics. The Oral Instruction Tantra contains many more chapters on specific diseases that are not covered here.

The third part is dedicated to therapeutics, with an emphasis on herbal treatment. "Herbal" is actually a misnomer, because many ingredients are also of animal and mineral origin. However, in order to avoid the frequent repetition of the more correct "medicinal ingredient" or "materia medica," the term *herb* was retained for brevity. While there remain problems with the identification of herbs, enough material can already be presented meaningfully. Some herbs are rather unknown outside the Himalayas. Further research will no doubt yield useful insights. However, many of the herbs used in Tibetan medicine, and in particular those most commonly used, are also well known to the Chinese, Indian, and Greco-Arabic traditional herbal systems. Indeed, the herbs were largely imported from their respective countries in the formative years of the medical system.[4] Some of the herbs are also well known in the European herbal tradition. A significant

---

[4.] Acknowledging the syncretic origins of Tibetan medicine does not preclude seeing the Medicine Buddha himself as its source, since according to Tibetan medicine all medical traditions are emanations of the Medicine Buddha.

amount of modern pharmacological research now exists for many of the "Tibetan" herbs. That research has been mostly the contribution of China, India, and Western countries since the latter half of the twentieth century. Appropriate references are therefore given as could be found. This book does not attempt to describe all of the Tibetan pharmacopoeia, as this would easily amount to thousands of herbs and other substances, but instead concentrates on the most commonly used must-know herbs and formulas. An enormous amount of time was spent recouping identifying information from available sources. In spite of that, there is still some ambiguity and uncertainty about a number of herbs. Accordingly, some of the herb identifications and naming styles are in disagreement with those of well-noted authors. Further discussion is welcome.

"Tibetan medicine" is far from uniform. There exist many related traditions that extend through the Himalayas and as far as Mongolia and Buryatia. It might more accurately be termed *amchi* medicine, this being the title given to its practitioners. Countless *amchis* have been trained through their respective family lineages or other apprenticeships rather than through standardized education. The practice also differs on the basis of locally available plants and other medicinals. There are endless possible variations, the vast majority of which may well claim to be authentic. The information presented in this book represents medical knowledge as explained by a Tibetan doctor who was recently trained in the Four Tantra tradition at *sman rtsis khang*.

There is still much more to Tibetan medicine. A great many chapters of the Four Tantras (much more than half) have not been translated except into Chinese, Mongolian, and Russian, and of course the question remains open whether those translations are usable if commentaries are not also available. Beyond the Four Tantras, there exists a vast body of Tibetan medical literature of great profundity that is almost entirely unknown in the West. Beyond this book, it might also be worth devising a practical manual to be used in the context of clinical training, describing moxibustion and bloodletting points, herb preparation, massage techniques, rejuvenation, jewel pills, etc. Time will tell whether the present authors will be privileged to write further works on Tibetan medicine. For now I am very grateful for the opportunity to make this small contribution to the art. I also wish to acknowledge Dr. Barry Clark and Dr. Barbara Gerke for their valuable review and advice.

ས་ཏ་མངྒ་ལོ།། ༎

May all beings be happy!

—Chris Hakim, May 2009

PART I

Review of Selected Topics

Being a Worthy Student

This part is based on the last chapter of the Fourth Tantra of Tibetan medicine. In this concluding chapter, the Tibetan doctor is instructed as to whom he or she should accept as a student of the art. Since Tibetan medicine is considered to be a Vajrayana Buddhist practice, this is especially important for both the teacher and the student. If the sacred knowledge of Tibetan medicine is misused or applied incorrectly, this entails a karmic liability not only for the student but also for the teacher, who is responsible for maintaining the integrity of the tradition. Since we inherit this tradition from the great doctors, visionaries, and teachers of the past, we are responsible for receiving it correctly and then passing it on unadulterated.

It is said that the milk of the white lioness is precious and exceedingly hard to obtain, and therefore should be held in a suitable container. Tibetan medicine likewise requires to be held, metaphorically, in the container of a student of suitable nature and disposition. Holding one's commitment to the lineage of medicine is seen as a vajra pledge, meaning holding the tradition in an authentic manner on penalty of negative karma. "Whoever is not a suitable recipient will not hold the vajra pledge." The chapter therefore contains warnings against teaching unsuitable students:

1. Those who, instead of appreciating the teacher, say they already know what they are being taught
2. Those who think they are better than the teacher
3. Those who, through cunning or deception, try to pry knowledge out of the teacher; or those who want to gain the teacher's favor through flattery but have no desire to help others
4. Those who would profit from any situation by deceiving others, always putting themselves first

One should be wary of such aspirants and hold all information from them in the same way a crocodile holds a jewel and does not let go. One should refuse to teach them even at the cost of one's life. One should not share knowledge with those who hold views contrary to the doctrine of wisdom and compassion.[5] On the other hand, the following qualities should be apparent in a worthy student:

1. Strong faith in the teacher
2. Boundless devotion, so that one would offer anything, even one's life, in order to learn

---

[5.] This is not meant to discourage non-Buddhists from studying Tibetan medicine.

3. Vast awareness: one's mind must be fully competent, so that the art may be learned fully, even if the teacher's knowledge is faulty at times.
4. Kindness
5. Altruism
6. A strong connection with the dharma, free of deceit

Another "set of six" is given in Chapter 31 of the Second Tantra, which describes the qualities of a good Tibetan doctor:

1. Intelligent
2. Altruistic
3. Adhering to his or her words of honor (*vajra* pledge)
4. Knowledgeable in practice
5. Diligent
6. Well versed in the social mores

Teaching such a qualified student is like placing the precious milk of the white lioness into a jeweled vessel.

THE HEALTHY BODY

The Internal Organs

Tibetan medicine regards the functions of internal organs empirically and met-aphorically. The functions ascribed to the organs do not correspond to modern findings, but nevertheless are part of a coherent and effective system of clinical reasoning that encompasses theory, observation, and treatment. This section reviews the main internal organs' metaphors and functions according to the physiology of traditional Tibetan medicine.

- The heart is responsible for the circulation of wind and blood. It is connected to the entire body's channels and blood vessels, especially the brain. It is like a king on his throne, ruling his kingdom from this central place.
- The five posterior lobes of the lungs are the king's closest ministers (advisors). The five anterior lobes are the king's princes. The function of the latter is to protect the king the way children protect their father.
- The liver and the spleen help digest the food by separating the pure part from the impure, thus producing blood. The liver is the king's senior consort, and the spleen his junior consort.
- The kidneys help develop the bodily constituents, protect the body from illness, purify the blood, strengthen the body, and sharpen the senses. They can be seen as the king's ministers at large, or as pillars that support the palace's central beam.
- The reproductive organs ensure reproduction and are seen as a treasury.
- The stomach receives food and drink and through the action of heat processes them for further digestion. It is like a cooking pot.
- The large and small intestines extract the pure part of nutrients and transfer it to the liver, while transferring the waste products as feces and urine. They are like the queen's attendants who serve meals and clean up afterward.
- The gallbladder assists in the digestive process by adding digestive heat. It is like a sac filled with spices that make food tender upon cooking.

The Process of Digestion

The life-sustaining wind is responsible for bringing food down to the stomach, where the watery and oily part of the food and drink ingested break up and soften all the materials. The fire-like wind then activates the digestive bile, which is likened to a boiling medicinal brew. The decomposing phlegm breaks the food down, making it sweeter. At that stage the phlegm humor increases. In a second phase, the digestive bile digests the food, making it sour, and the bile humor increases. Finally the fire-like wind digests the food and separates the pure part from the turbid, thus creating a bitter taste. At that stage the wind humor increases. The waste products of digestion are separated in the small intestine, where the liquid part is transformed into urine and the solid part into stool. The resulting chyme (the pure part of ingested food and drink, also called chyle, nutriment, etc.) is send to the liver, beginning the metabolic cycle of the seven bodily constituents.

The Seven Bodily Constituents

- Once food is ingested, it is metabolized into constituents of increasing refinement from chyme all the way to reproductive fluid as follows:
- Chyme is produced by the stomach as the end result of the digestive process, while the waste products of food and drink are excreted. Chyme is transferred to the liver, where it is refined into blood. The waste product of this refining process becomes phlegm.
- Blood moistens the body and sustains life. It is transformed into muscle tissue by the color-transforming bile. The waste product of that transformation becomes gall.
- The function of muscle is to cover the body. It is further refined into fat, while the residue becomes skin.
- Fat lubricates the body. Its purified product is bone, and the waste product of that transformation turns into the oiliness of various parts of the body.
- Bones support the body. Their refined product is marrow and the unrefined counterpart makes up teeth, nails, and body hair.
- Marrow produces nutriment essential to the body. Its refined part becomes reproductive fluid, while the unrefined part provides the oiliness of skin and stool.
- Reproductive fluid is responsible for conception. Its unrefined product is sperm or ovum and its refined product is vital fluid.

Vital fluid is the ultimate essence of all bodily constituents. It enters the blood so as to become inseparable from its pure essence. From the heart, vital fluid spreads through the entire body, promoting longevity, clarity of the senses, and radiance. It circulates through the body in daily, monthly, and yearly cycles and also changes through an individual's lifetime. This vital fluid belongs to the triad of channels, wind, and vital fluid, and it is the basis of advanced tantric practices (Thubten Phuntsog 2001).

The Three Excretions

The excretions are feces, urine, and perspiration. They are understood as processing more than just substance. In this way the feces' function is seen as supporting the decomposition and evacuation of ingested food. The urine supports the body fluids and assists in their transformation and excretion. The sweat softens the skin and unblocks the pores.

The Humors as Normal Bodily Functions

In the correct state of balance the three humors, wind, bile, and phlegm, perform normal bodily functions. Each humor is divided into five functional subtypes.

Wind

Wind normally resides in the waist and hips and generally in the lower part of the body. It is responsible for respiration, movement, excretion, clarity of the senses, and sustenance of the body. The nature of wind is coarse, light, cold, subtle, hard, and mobile. The pathways of wind disorders are the bones, ears, channels, heart, life channel, and large intestine.

Subdivisions of Wind

- The life-sustaining wind resides at the crown of the head and circulates in the throat and sternum. It is responsible for swallowing, inhalation, salivation, sneezing, eructation, clarity of the mind and sense organs, and unity of the body and mind. It is also responsible for the formation of the embryo and is the source of the four other kinds of wind.
- The ascending wind resides at the chest and circulates in the nose, tongue, and throat. It is responsible for speech, physical strength, radiance, complexion, diligence, and memory.
- The pervasive wind resides at the heart and circulates throughout the body. It is responsible for movement, opening and closing of the orifices, and most other physical, verbal, and mental activity.
- The fire-like wind resides in the stomach and circulates in the digestive tract. It is responsible for digestion, specifically the separation between chyme and waste products, and provides nourishment to the body.
- The purgative wind is located in the perineum or sacrum and circulates in the large intestine, bladder, genitals, and thighs. It is responsible for parturition and for the retention and discharge of semen, sexual fluids, menstrual blood, stool, and urine.

Bile

Bile normally resides around the diaphragm and generally in the middle part of the body. It is responsible for the feeling of hunger and thirst, digestion, bodily heat, clarity of complexion, courage, and intelligence. The nature of bile is oily, sharp, hot, light, malodorous, laxative, and moist. The pathways of bile disorders are the blood, sweat, eyes, liver, gallbladder, and small intestine.

Subdivisions of Bile

- The digestive bile resides at the interface between digested and undigested matter (this may mean in the small intestine). It is responsible for digestion, body heat, and vigor, and it assists the other four kinds of bile.
- The color-transforming bile resides in the liver. It is responsible for the coloring of the bodily constituents and excretions.
- The accomplishing bile resides in the heart. It is responsible for discrimination, pride, and diligence in accomplishing one's aims.
- The vision-producing bile resides in the eyes and is responsible for vision.
- The complexion-clearing bile resides in the skin. It is responsible for maintaining a healthy complexion.

Phlegm

Phlegm normally resides in the brain and generally in the upper part of the body. It is responsible for firmness of mind and body, sleep, joint lubrication, patience, and smoothness of the skin. The nature of phlegm is oily, cool, heavy, blunt, smooth, firm, steady, and viscous. The pathways of phlegm are chyme, muscle, fat, marrow, reproductive fluids, stool, urine, the nose, tongue, lungs, spleen, stomach, kidneys, and bladder.

Subdivisions of Phlegm

- The supporting phlegm resides in the chest. It assists the four other kinds of phlegm and maintains the body's moisture.
- The decomposing phlegm resides in the stomach. It decomposes and churns the food and liquids ingested.
- The gustatory phlegm resides in the tongue. It is responsible for the sense of taste.
- The satisfying phlegm resides in the head. It aids all the sense organs and thus produces sensory acuity.
- The connective phlegm resides in all the joints and is responsible for their suppleness.

Two Flowers and Three Fruits

The two flowers of the healthy body are freedom from disease and longevity. Those give rise to the three fruits, which are spiritual achievement, wealth, and lasting happiness.

ILLNESS AND ITS INVESTIGATION

Causes of Disease

Primary Causes

Tibetan medicine posits that all disease arises in relation to the mind in one way or another. Obviously external physical factors and events (environmental exposure, injury, etc.) intervene too, but they are seen as the result of karma, which is the sum total of an individual's good and bad past actions. Thus even seemingly external events are the result of volitional action, which arises in the individual's mind, be that an action performed in this life or in a previous life. Buddhist doctrine holds the three factors of desire, hatred, and ignorance as the root psychological factors that lead to negative action and therefore karmic liability. These three factors, called the three poisons of the mind, originate from *ma rig pa,* or fundamental ignorance. In this way, the primary cause of wind disorders is desire. The primary cause of bile disorders is hatred or anger. The primary cause of phlegm disorders is ignorance or confusion.

The doctrine of karma is often described in the West as fatalistic because it seems to lead its adherents simply to accept their fate. In fact, Buddhist teachings offer many methods for purifying karma, such as performing good deeds, living with contentment, and cultivating a conducive state of mind. Far from making their practitioners feel powerless, the teachings of the Buddha invite people to take responsibility for their actions and for the world.

Secondary Causes

Secondary causes are the seasons, environment, age, lifestyle, and diet, which are described below. Disturbances caused by elemental provocations are also described in the Four Tantras.

Entry Modes of Disease

Disease spreads through the skin, expands in the muscles, circulates through the channels and blood vessels, attaches itself to the bones, descends onto the solid organs, and finally flows through the hollow organs. Refer to the chapters on each humor for more details.

Location and Pathways of the Humors

Wind

Wind resides in the lower part of the body, especially the pelvis. Its pathological manifestations are mainly in the bones, ears, pores of the skin, heart, blood vessels, channels, and large intestine.

Bile

Bile resides in the middle part of the body, especially the liver and gallbladder. It manifests as disease in the blood, sweat, eyes, liver, gallbladder, and small intestine.

Phlegm

Phlegm resides in the upper part of the body, especially the brain. It manifests as disease in the chyme, muscles, fat, marrow, reproductive fluids, feces, urine, nose, tongue, lungs, spleen, kidneys, stomach, and bladder.

Summary

In summary, all diseases are hot or cold by nature. Cold diseases are associated with phlegm. Hot diseases are associated with blood and bile. Wind, although of cold nature, can be associated with both heat and cold and thus is the root of all disease and accompanies it throughout. Therefore, close attention is always paid to wind in the treatment of illness.

Interrogation and Examination

Although the tongue, pulse, and urine are reliable diagnostic indicators, the doctor should not fail to ask the patient about causative dietary and lifestyle factors, ask about or look for appropriate signs and symptoms and inquire about ameliorating factors. In case of doubt, exploratory treatment can be given, for example bone broth if a wind condition is suspected, in order to obtain unambiguous information about the patient's condition.

Causative Personal, Dietary, Lifestyle, and Environmental Factors

The factors of diet, lifestyle, age, and environment that lead to humoral imbalance can be categorized thus:

- Wind: old age, light, rough foods, rough lifestyle, and a cold windy environment

- Bile: adulthood, sharp pungent foods, sitting in the sun or other dry or hot places, strenuous physical activity
- Phlegm: childhood, heavy greasy food, and sitting or lying on grass, dirt, or other cold and humid environments

Signs and Symptoms

The cardinal signs and symptoms of humoral imbalance are the following:

- Wind: yawning, shivering, stretching, moving pains in the joints, dullness of the senses, mental instability, sensation of hunger, and worsening of the symptoms during summer, at dawn, and in the afternoon
- Bile: bitter taste in the mouth, sensations of heat over the skin, pain in the upper part of the body, headache, pain after digestion, and worsening of the symptoms in autumn, at noon, and at midnight
- Phlegm: poor appetite, poor digestion, belching, sensation of heaviness, cold extremities, internal sensation of cold, discomfort after eating, and worsening of the symptoms in the spring, in the morning, and in the evening

Ameliorating Factors

It is often helpful to query the patient as to the factors that may give rise to improvement or alleviation, with the following guidelines to identify the corresponding humor:

- Wind: oily and nourishing foods, resting in warm places, enjoying the company of friends, and gentle music
- Bile: cooling diets and staying in cool places
- Phlegm: warming foods, wearing warm clothing, and staying in warm places

The doctor may also resort to exploratory treatment in order to ascertain the nature of an illness. For example, if the patient benefits from taking bone broth, this may confirm a wind disorder, and a positive result from taking a decoction of *tig ta* (chiretta) would indicate a bile disorder.

Pulse Diagnosis

The pulse is caused by the wind pushing the blood through the blood vessels. Since wind governs the entire body, sensing the pulse gives a reflection of the whole body's state of health. Reading the pulse is subtle, complex, and hard to master. This skill is best acquired in a clinical setting though systematic practice and observation.

Taking the Pulse

Prior to having his or her pulse examined, the patient should refrain from certain foods and drinks that might interfere by mimicking various illnesses:

- Coffee, very strong tea, goat meat, pork, or fasting, excessive talking, sex, lack of sleep, and stressful activity should be avoided in order not to create an impression of a wind disorder.
- Meat, alcohol, and other excessively hot substances, or eating and drinking to excess, should be avoided in order not to create an impression of a hot disorder.
- Stale, cold, and unripe foods could mimic a phlegm disorder and should likewise be avoided.

The physician should likewise be fully available for taking the pulse, being well rested, and having refrained from alcohol, sex, and strenuous or stressful activity prior to examining the patient. The best time for taking the pulse is in the morning.

The pulse is taken by applying the index, middle, and ring fingers of both hands on the patient's radial arteries at both wrists. The index fingers are pressed lightly to feel the skin, the middle fingers moderately to feel the flesh, and the ring fingers strongly to feel the bone. Each finger position represents two organs, depending on the side of the fingertip that feels the pulse. The distal side with respect to the patient represents a solid organ, while the proximal side of the fingertip represents a hollow organ, according to the figure below. The index finger positions have the organs reversed between male and female patients.

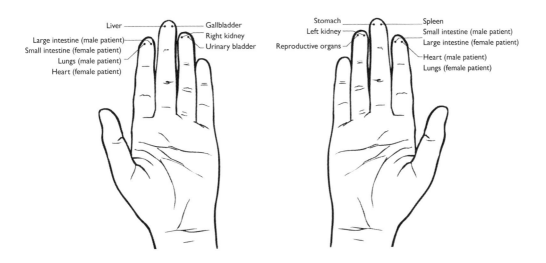

Basic Pulse Patterns

The basic pulse presentations for humoral imbalances are:

- Wind: floating and empty on pressure
- Bile: fast, thin, and taut; prominent and palpable even when pressed
- Phlegm: slow, sunken, weak, and indistinct

Complex Pulse Images

Complex disorders produce specific pulse images (Tenzing Dakpa 2007). These are common examples:

- Wind and fever: empty and fast
- Bile and phlegm: sunken and taut
- Wind and phlegm: empty and slow
- Dark phlegm: thick and full, weak under the middle fingers
- Blood disorder: bounding and rolling
- Lymph disorder: trembling, slow, and hesitant
- High fever: strong and taut but rolling when pressed
- Chronic fever: thin and taut

Many more pulse-diagnosis techniques have been presented elsewhere. These include seasonal and elemental influences, pregnancy, the patient's life force (*bla*), evil spirits, death, and other forms of prognostication, not all of which are mastered uniformly by all Tibetan physicians (Tenzing Dakpa 2007).

Urine Diagnosis

Diagnosis by examination of the patient's urine is another important diagnostic method fairly unique to the Tibetan medical system. Like pulse diagnosis, it requires much skill and attentiveness to produce accurate results.

Collecting and Examining the Urine

As for pulse diagnosis, the patient should refrain from certain food, drink, and activities that might affect the urine and thus produce misleading results. The best time to collect urine is in the morning, as long as the patient voided urine the previous night to eliminate the influence of the previous day's diet and activities. The urine should be caught midstream. The best time to examine the urine is also the morning, when the sun gives the best light. Daylight should be used for better color accuracy. The urine should be poured into a clean container with a white bottom so that the color will be seen clearly. After the urine has settled in the container, sediment may form at the bottom. This is representative of the state of the blood and bile in the patient's body.

Diagnostic Criteria

Healthy Urine

Healthy urine should be light yellow, form medium-sized bubbles when stirred, and form a moderate amount of sediment at the bottom and a moderate amount of film on the surface. Its color should change to pale yellow after stirring has stopped.

The Humors Reflected in the Urine

Urine present in humoral imbalance differs from healthy urine in the following ways:

- Wind: watery and bluish with large bubbles forming on stirring
- Bile: reddish yellow, strong smelling, with a lot of fume and small bubbles that disappear rapidly after stirring
- Phlegm: whitish and turbid with little smell or fume, and many bubbles forming on stirring that stay on the surface like saliva

Heat and Cold Reflected in the Urine

The urine can be analyzed in further detail by noting changes in film and sediment when the urine has cooled down somewhat, and changes in turbidity when the urine has become cold:

- Urine in hot conditions has a strong yellow color with abundant film sediment and fume as it cools down. When the urine is cold, it changes from clear to turbid.
- Urine that indicates cold illness has a pale or whitish color with little or no film sediment or fume as it cools down. When the urine is cold, it changes from turbid to clear.

Sometimes the urine presents a contradictory picture where the color indicates cold but the amount of sediment suggests heat, or vice versa. In both cases the amount of sediment governs the diagnosis:

- If the urine is whitish-blue with a lot of sediment, this may indicate a deep-seated hot disorder.

- If the urine is reddish-yellow with light odor and no sediment, this may indicate a cold disorder.

If the amount of bubbles does not accord with the other characteristics of the urine, the other characteristics (color, fume, etc.) take precedence:

- If the urine is reddish-yellow with no bubbles, this may indicate a deeply-buried hot disorder.
- If the urine is whitish or bluish with no bubbles, this may indicate chronic cold.

Like the pulse, the urine has also been used as a means of prognostication of death, evil spirits, etc. A much more detailed description of Tibetan urinalysis has been published elsewhere (Lobsang Rapgay 1985; Tenzing Dakpa 2007).

Tongue Diagnosis

The basic tongue presentations for humoral imbalance are:

- Wind: red, dry, and rough, with or without cracks
- Bile: covered with a thick pale-yellow coat
- Phlegm: dull, smooth, and moist, with a sticky coat

Patterns of Disease in the Tongue

Complex disorders produce specific tongue presentations (Tenzing Dakpa 2007). Here are common examples:

- Void fever: dry, rough, and black at the center
- High bile fever: black at the center and a bitter taste in the patient's mouth
- Heat in the blood: dry and red
- Wind and bile combined disorder: yellow, dry, and stiff
- Wind and phlegm combined disorder: pale, dry, and stiff
- Dark phlegm: brown with cracks
- Fever caused by dark phlegm: dry, stiff, with a bitter taste in the patient's mouth
- Spread fever: pale, thickened, and dull
- Unripe fever: pale with small red dots
- Fever affecting the heart: blackened tip
- Heart disorder: cracks at the center
- Kidney disorder: black bands on the sides

Miscellaneous Diagnostic Techniques

Other diagnostic techniques involve examination of the complexion, eyes, nose, lips, sputum, feces, vomitus, blood, etc. Analysis of a person's constitutional type (wind, bile, phlegm, or a combination) also helps understand their propensity to illness. All those methods and criteria have been explained elsewhere (Tenzing Dakpa 2007) and need not be restated.

Prognosis: Nine Factors of Fatal Outcome

There exist nine factors that indicate a poor prognosis, incurability, and possibly even death:

1. Exhaustion of the three factors that sustain life: the life span, merit, and one's karma (the exhaustion of one's natural life span, the exhaustion of one's merit, and sudden unexpected death [Tenzing Dakpa 2007])
2. A fatal combination of hot and cold humors such that treating one makes the other worse and vice versa
3. Prior treatment of a cold disease with a cold remedy or treatment of a hot disease with a hot remedy
4. Injury to one of the body's vulnerable points (one of the 45 points of the flesh, 8 points of the fat, 32 points of the bones, etc. as described in Chapter 4 of the Explanatory or Second Tantra)
5. Delayed treatment of a wind disorder, resulting in the decline of the ascending wind, which is itself the support for the life-sustaining wind
6. Delayed treatment of a fever disorder
7. Delayed treatment of a deep-seated cold disorder
8. Depletion of the bodily constituents, making the patient unresponsive to treatment
9. Serious injury by elemental spirits, causing loss of the patient's life force (bla)

PART II

The Humors

DISORDERS CAUSED BY WIND

This chapter is derived from the second chapter of the Oral Instruction Tantra and related sources. The fact that this chapter appears in the Oral Instruction Tantra as the first detailed description of disease emphasizes the importance of wind in the causation of all other illnesses. As is said at the end of the chapter, ascites, edema, anemia, nausea, and hidden tumors originate from the accumulation of the disturbed humors, for all of which wind is the guiding factor. It is said that wind is parasitic by nature. It easily pervades the body, thus causing harm and bringing forth diseases, including those of bile and phlegm. This means that wind can be hot or cold, depending on it combining with other humors.

According to the Buddhist view, there are three fundamental mental afflictions: passion or desire, anger or hatred, and ignorance or delusion. Those three afflictions or poisons are said to arise from basic ignorance of the true nature of reality. Of the three poisons, passion is the fundamental cause of wind disease.

Immediate Causes

Since wind is rough and light by nature, similar conditions exacerbate it: excessive intake of bitter, light, or rough foods or of nonnutritious foods; drinking cold water in excess; excessive sexual intercourse; irregular eating or sleeping; persistent hunger or undernourishment; excessive physical, mental, or verbal activity, especially on an empty stomach; severe diarrhea or vomiting; blood loss; exposure to cold wind; excessive grief, melancholy, or depression; forced retention or expulsion of stool, sperm, or urine; etc. When these causes meet with other factors, such as the season or bodily constitution, which are also causative of wind conditions, wind conditions are sure to arise.

The contemporary reader will not fail to recognize those causative factors as typical of the modern lifestyle: having a lot of different activities throughout the day, time pressures, fast food instead of an adequate diet, lack of sleep, not enough time to relax, etc. We are all familiar with patterns of boundless ambition, mental agitation, hypertension, insomnia, rapid emotional changes, depression, and so forth. Wind also often manifests as post-traumatic stress disorder (PTSD), as is often seen in displaced populations and other patients who have gone through great upheavals.

General Diagnosis of Wind Disorders

The general signs and symptoms of wind disorders are:

- Pulse: empty and floating, with changing rate or skipped beats
- Urine: clear and bluish, with large bubbles and no steam, sediment, or smell
- Tongue: dry, reddish, and rough
- Mental and nervous factors: vertigo, delirium, irritability, insomnia, sighing, and yawning
- Surface of the body: chills, cracked skin, a sensation of being bound, goose bumps, pain on wearing clothes, and a feeling of the skin being torn away
- Neuromuscular symptoms: cramps in the extremities, impaired flexion or extension of the limbs, soreness as if beaten up, and frequent stretching
- Pain: in the neck, chest, or temples, diffused or intermittent pain, sharp pain on moving, and pain at the wind points (the first, sixth, and seventh vertebrae[6] or C7, T5 and T6, respectively)
- Other indications: astringent taste in the mouth, tinnitus, lassitude, nausea without vomiting, abdominal rumble, and flatulence

Aggravation of the above occurs in the early morning, late afternoon, and after digestion.

Diagnosis sometimes needs to be clarified by exploratory treatment or by investigating ameliorating and aggravating factors. If the intake of meat, alcohol, *bu ram* (raw cane sugar), old butter or ghee, or any hot food and drink improves the patient's condition, or if the patient's condition improves after undergoing a generic treatment of wind disorders (see the next section), then a wind condition is indicated. Likewise, if the patient's condition is made worse by exposure to cold, eating cold foods, excessive sexual intercourse or strenuous exercise, lack of sleep, etc., this also suggests a wind disorder.

General Treatment of Wind Disorders

The treatments offered in this section are beneficial for all wind disorders and are generally sufficient if the condition is not severe or complicated by other factors. Such generic treatments can also be applied to confirm a tentative diagnosis of wind.

[6.] Vertebrae are counted differently in the Tibetan and Western medical systems.

Lifestyle and Diet

The patient should wear warm clothes, reside in a warm pleasant place that is free of disturbance or excessive demands, and enjoy the company of pleasant people. The diet should be nutritious or even rich but easy to digest. Foods especially recommended for wind conditions include radish, garlic, onion, baked dough, mutton, soup of sheep bones, old butter or ghee, *bu ram* (raw cane sugar), dried meat, sesame oil, fresh milk, and a moderate amount of mild grain beer. If lifestyle and dietary changes are not sufficient, the general remedies below can be helpful.

Bone Soup

Traditionally, three kinds of bones are used: ankle, scapula, and sacrum, preferably of sheep. Meat soup can be supplemented with *bu ram* (raw cane sugar) and alcohol or with *dzA ti* (nutmeg), *kha ru tshwa* (black salt), *shing kun* (asafetida), *sman sga* (ginger), *sgog skya* (garlic), *go snyod* (caraway), and other substances that treat wind.

Alcoholic Preparations

These are usually based on mild grain beer mixed with *bu ram* (raw cane sugar), cereals, *gze ma* (puncture vine), *lca ba* (angelica), *ra mnye* (Solomon's seal), and other nutritious substances that treat wind.

Soups That Expel Wind *('don)*

There are four types, called white soup (dkar 'don), red soup (dmar 'don), sour soup (skyur 'don), and garlic soup (sgog 'don):

- White soup: sesame oil and thsom phye (a paste of roasted barley flour with milk cooked together) boiled in milk with *sman sga* (ginger) and *rgyam tshwa* (rock salt)
- Red soup: the above with mutton added
- Sour soup: a preparation made of fermented rice, old butter or ghee, *bu ram* (raw cane sugar) and *sman sga* (ginger)
- Garlic soup: a preparation made of garlic paste, old butter or ghee, bone soup, and *rgyam tshwa* (rock salt)

Medicinal Powder

A medicinal powder should be made with one part each of *dzA ti* (nutmeg), *shing kun* (asafetida), *kha ru tshwa* (black salt), *rgyam tshwa* (rock salt), *rtsab ru tshwa* (crag halite), *sman sga* (ginger), *pi pi ling* (long pepper), *na le sham* (black pepper), *shing tsha* (cinnamon), *se 'bru* (pomegranate), *sug smel* (green cardamom), *a ru ra* (chebulic myrobalan), *sle tres* (moonseed), *sgog skya* (garlic), and eight parts of *ka ra* (white rock sugar) or *bu ram* (raw cane sugar).

If cold is predominant, the dosage of *shing kun* (asafetida) should be doubled, while if heat is predominant, the dosage of *dzA ti* (nutmeg) should be doubled. This powder should be given together with one of the soups described above.

Medicinal Butter

All medicinal-butter recipes below are applicable to general wind disorders. Some also have specific applications.

- Medicinal butter with *sgog skya* (garlic) and *bu ram* (raw cane sugar) as a general treatment
- Medicinal butter with *ra mnye* (Solomon's seal), *nye shing* (asparagus), *lca ba* (angelica), *ba spru* (Himalayan mirabilis), and *gze ma* (puncture vine) as general treatment
- Medicinal butter with *bong nga dkar po* (white aconite), crushed bones, *a ru ra* (chebulic myrobalan), *ba ru ra* (beleric myrobalan), *skyu ru ra* (amla), *ra mnye* (Solomon's seal), *nye shing* (asparagus), *lca ba* (angelica), *ba spru* (Himalayan mirabilis), and *gze ma* (puncture vine) as a general treatment
- Medicinal butter with *a ru ra* (chebulic myrobalan), *ba ru ra* (beleric myrobalan), and *skyu ru ra* (amla) as a general treatment
- Medicinal butter with *kha ru tshwa* (black salt), *pi pi ling* (long pepper), and *a ru ra* (chebulic myrobalan) when the upper part of the body is affected
- Medicinal butter with *se 'bru* (pomegranate), *'u su* (coriander), *sman sga* (ginger), *tsi tra ka* (wild leadwort), and *pi pi ling* (long pepper) to improve the appetite and digestion and to improve muscle tone

In summary, preparation begins by boiling the herbs first in water and reducing the liquid slightly. The herbs are then removed, and milk is added to the liquid. When the volume of liquid has been reduced to that of the milk alone, the same volume of butter is added. The liquid is then boiled until all moisture has been evaporated and the liquid becomes oily. This is tested by listening to the sound made by throwing a small amount of liquid onto fire. When the preparation cools down, powdered herbs similar to those decocted and equal parts of *bu ram* (raw cane sugar), *ka ra* (white rock sugar), and *sbrang rtsi* (honey) are added. Honey must be purified by first boiling it in water with a small piece of goat meat. The process is complete when the meat changes color, at which time the meat should be removed and discarded. The preparation of medicinal butter employs very low heat and typically takes several hours.

Other Modalities for the Treatment of Wind

Other modalities include enema, fumigation, inhalation, massage, and poultices, all of which are described at the end of the section on therapeutics.

Classification and Treatment by Type of Illness

Wind disorders can be loosely classified into the following eight broad categories: stiffness, contraction, atrophy, swelling, contraction or deviation, pain, delirium, and loss of consciousness. Expanded categories follow in the rest of this section with slightly different headings, as per the original text.

Convulsions

Convulsions should be treated by inhalation therapy and by pouring warm sesame oil into the patient's ear. Any of the nourishing foods described at the beginning of the chapter can be beneficial.

A medicated fat suitable for massage, fomentation, enema, etc. can be made with the four types of fat (oil, old butter or ghee, meat fat, and bone marrow) boiled with *shug pa tsher* can (juniper), sgron shing (pine node), *sle tres* (moonseed), *lca ba* (angelica), *ba spru* (Himalayan mirabilis), *ra mnye* (Solomon's seal), *gze ma* (puncture vine), *nye shing* (asparagus), *ru rta* (costus), *rgya spos* (clover), *kaNDa ka ri* (two-flowered raspberry), meat soup, milk, *bu ram* (raw cane sugar), and drink made from fermented *bu ram* (raw cane sugar).

The "Bending" Disorders

The "bending" disorders can be treated by means of inhalation therapy or massage over the head and eyes with sesame oil, as well as by pouring sesame oil into the ears. If there is edema, emesis (described in the chapter on phlegm) and bloodletting should also be performed.

"Forward Bending"

Forward bending of the body, sighing, exhaustion, mental confusion, bulging eyes, breathing difficulty, muscle wasting, weight loss, stiffness of the spine

"Backward Bending"

Backward bending of the body, prominent chest, clenched teeth, frothy saliva, disturbed speech, pain in the jaw, neck, and back, bulging eyes, yawning, pain in the rib cage, loose joints

"Inward Bending"

Similar to the "backward bending" syndrome

"Sideways Bending"

Facial paralysis, bending on one side of the body, deviation of the mouth or jaw, bulging eyes, amnesia, fright on waking up

Stiffness of the Thighs

Signs and symptoms are severe pain in the legs due to infiltration of phlegm, loss of sensation in the legs, loss of body heat, impaired motion, and sensation of heaviness of the legs. Stiffness of the thigh is caused by impaired digestion *(ma zhu)*, phlegm, and excess fat.

- The following decoction should be given: *gu gul* (myrrh), *brag zhun* (mineral pitch), and *a ru ra* (chebulic myrobalan) together with cow urine.
- This powder can also be given: *gla sgang* (bistort), *tsi tra ka* (wild leadwort), *sman sga* (ginger), *pi pi ling* (long pepper), *na le sham* (black pepper), *gu gul* (myrrh), *a ru ra* (chebulic myrobalan), *ba ru ra* (beleric myrobalan), *skyu ru ra* (amla), and *byi tang ga* (false black pepper).
- Physical exercise is also recommended for this condition.

Paralysis, Lameness, and Sciatica

- Paralysis of the shoulder: limitation of movement and loss of sensation in the arm
- Paralysis of the forearm: stiffness or limitation of movement in the forearm, wrist, and hand
- Lameness: looseness of the joints, wobbling or limping gait, leg tremors or jerking movements
- Hemiplegia: paralysis, loss of sensation or severe pain in half of the body
- Paraplegia: weight loss, muscle wasting and paralysis, loss of sensation or severe pain in the entire body
- Sciatica: progressive stiffening of the heel, calf, and thigh

Treatment: give the powder of *pi pi ling* gi rtsa ba (root of the long-pepper plant), *dong gra* (lesser galangal), *tsi tra ka* (wild leadwort), *pi pi ling* (long pepper), and *ma nu pa tra* (elecampane); this recipe can also be prepared as a medicinal butter. Sciatica and paralysis of the forearm can also be treated by bloodletting.

Malfunction of the Blood Vessels of the Head and Stiffness of the Whole Body

- Malfunction of the blood vessels of the head: discoloration of the top of the head at the suture of the skull, impaired senses
- Stiffness of the whole body: limited flexion or extension of the extremities, stiffness of the entire body; this condition entails a loss of assimilation of food with subsequent phlegm.

These conditions can be treated by giving a mixture of *rgya spos* (clover), *ru rta* (costus), *sug smel* (green cardamom), *shu dag nag po* (sweet flag), *shu dag dkar po* (Japanese sweet flag), *tsan dan dmar po* (red sandalwood), *rdo dreg* (salted shield), *spang spos* (muskroot), *'u su nag po* (black coriander), sesame oil, *ka ra* (white rock sugar), and old butter or ghee. This recipe is applicable to all wind disorders and also treats insanity, hidden tumors, and swollen testicles *(rlig rlugs).*[7]

Miscellaneous Types of Wind Disorders

Several other wind conditions are described in the Oral Instruction Tantra without specific treatment:

- Lockjaw or atrophy of the jaw: the mouth remains open or closed, causing difficulty speaking, eating, and drinking.
- Stiffness of the tongue: slurred speech, inability to move the tongue, difficulty eating and drinking
- Swelling of the knees: swelling of the knees, thickening of the skin
- Pain and stiffness of the ankles
- Spasm of the fingers and toes
- Tingling sensation in the feet: burning or stinging sensation in the legs as caused by wind and phlegm
- Burning sensation in the soles of the feet, especially when walking

Classification and Treatment by Location

The location of a wind condition progresses along with the severity of the illness. Thus the wind at first gets lodged in the skin, enters the channels, attaches itself to the bones, spreads to the solid organs, falls upon the hollow organs, and finally "blossoms" in the sense organs (head, eyes, eyes, ears, nose, and tongue). Detailed classification and treatment of wind disorders are presented in the rest of this section.

---

[7] This may correspond to inguinal hernia.

Wind Affecting the Skin

Symptoms: pain, tingling or rough sensation on the skin, or a sensation that the skin is cracked

Treatment consists of massage with sesame oil and a diet that includes bone soup.

Wind Affecting the Muscles, Fat, Tendons, Ligaments, Joints, and Blood Vessels

- Wind affecting the muscles: pimples, dryness or roughness of the skin, swelling, discoloration
- Wind affecting the fat: loss of appetite, swelling
- Wind affecting the tendons and ligaments: paralysis, stiffness, or weakness of the limbs
- Wind affecting the joints: loose and swollen joints
- Wind affecting the blood vessels: swelling of the blood vessels, blood vessels feeling empty to the touch

All these conditions are treated by massage and the application of warm ointments.

Wind Affecting the Bones or the Bone Marrow

- Wind affecting the bones: pain in the joints or in the bones, weight loss, exhaustion
- Wind affecting the bone marrow: insomnia and a sensation of being bandaged tightly, which is relieved by pressure or massage

These two conditions are treated by giving nutritious food, massage, and an enema made of the four kinds of fat (sesame oil, old butter or ghee, meat fat, and bone marrow).

Wind Affecting the Semen

Signs and symptoms: watery or lumpy semen

This condition is usually related to old age and is therefore treated by means of rejuvenation therapy. For this purpose, medicinal butter should be made with *da byid smug po* (stream salamander), *lca ba* (angelica), *ba spru* (Himalayan mirabilis), *ra mnye* (Solomon's seal), *gze ma* (puncture vine), *nye shing* (asparagus), *a ru ra* (chebulic myrobalan), *ba ru ra* (beleric myrobalan), *skyu ru ra* (amla), *bre ga* (pennycress), and sheep testicle. The medicinal butter should be mixed with *rgya tshwa* (ammonium chloride), *sug smel* (green cardamom), *bca' sga* (fresh ginger), and *pi pi ling* (long pepper), and then kept covered in whole grain, such as wheat or barley, for three to four weeks. (Covering with grain is the traditional Tibetan way of keeping fruit until it ripens.)

Wind Affecting the Blood

Signs and symptoms: sleepiness, redness of the blood vessels, skin discoloration

Treat by massage with the application of fat. This should be followed by the appropriate bloodletting therapy. If there is numbness as a result of the bloodletting, apply sesame oil mixed with soot from a wood-burning oven or a butter lamp and *rgyam tshwa* (rock salt) over the wind points.

Wind Affecting the Heart

Signs and symptoms: mental agitation, sighing

- Treatment: decoction of *sman sga* (ginger) and *shing kun* (asafetida), with *rgyam tshwa* (rock salt) added after boiling
- Medicinal butter made with *a ru ra* (chebulic myrobalan), *ba ru ra* (beleric myrobalan), and *skyu ru ra* (amla) is also effective.

Wind Affecting the Liver

Signs and symptoms: yawning when hungry, sensation of sagging of the liver

- Give the patient liver sizzled with spices in a bronze pan.
- *kha ru tshwa* (black salt), *gur gum* (safflower), and *brag zhun* (mineral pitch) may also be given.
- A medicinal bath made of different kinds of bones is also beneficial.
- Moxibustion is indicated.

Wind Affecting the Spleen

Signs and symptoms: swelling, abdominal distention or rumbling, indigestion, flatulence

Treat with *sman sga* (ginger), *pi pi ling* (long pepper), and *na le sham* (black pepper) mixed with old butter or ghee.

Wind Affecting the Kidneys

Signs and symptoms: lumbar pain, diminished hearing

- The chief remedy for this condition is *gze ma* (puncture vine) decocted and fermented into wine.
- Different kinds of nutritious soups containing *bu ram* (raw cane sugar) are helpful.
- Medicinal butter made with *ra mnye* (Solomon's seal), *nye shing* (asparagus), *lca ba* (angelica), *ba spru* (Himalayan mirabilis), and *gze ma* (puncture vine) may also be taken for this condition.
- Moxibustion is indicated.

Wind Affecting the Lungs

Signs and symptoms: swelling of the face, cough with or without mucus

Treat with *star bu* (sea buckthorn), *cu gang* (bamboo pith), *zi ra dkar po* (cumin), and *sug smel* (green cardamom).

Wind Affecting All the Solid Organs

This condition is treated by means of moxibustion.

Wind Affecting the Stomach

Signs and symptoms: discomfort in the stomach and throughout the body, aggravated after meals

- This condition is treated with the powder of *se 'bru* (pomegranate), *shing tsha* (cinnamon), *dzA ti* (nutmeg), *sug smel* (green cardamom), *ka ko la* (black cardamom), *rgya tshwa* (ammonium chloride), *rgyam tshwa* (rock salt), *kha ru tshwa* (black salt), *zi ra dkar po* (cumin), *zi ra nag po* (fennelflower), *sman sga* (ginger), *pi pi ling* (long pepper), *na le sham* (black pepper), and la la phud mixed with *bu ram* (raw cane sugar) steeped in wine.
- Moxibustion is indicated.

Wind Affecting the Small Intestine

Signs and symptoms: belching, vomiting, loss of appetite, abdominal distention, intestinal rumbling, thirst, shortness of breath

Treat by emesis (described in the chapter on phlegm) followed by foods and drugs that stimulate digestion.

Wind Affecting the Large Intestine

Signs and symptoms: colicky pain, flatulence, intestinal rumbling, constipation, scant urination, pain in the lumbar and sacral regions

- Treat by enema.
- The patient should also be given medicinal butter made with *sgog skya* (garlic) to take before meals.
- The following herb combination can also be helpful: *se 'bru* (pomegranate), *rgya tshwa* (ammonium chloride), *rgyam tshwa* (rock salt), *kha ru tshwa* (black salt), and *bu ram* (raw cane sugar).
- Moxibustion is indicated.

Wind Affecting the Gallbladder

Signs and symptoms: swelling and pain in the liver and gallbladder area, indigestion, jaundice, cataract

- Give the patient powder of *'jam 'bras* (fever nut), *gser gyi me tog* (bolenggua), *tig ta* (chiretta) and *rgyam tshwa* (rock salt). This powder stimulates the power of digestion.
- Moxibustion is indicated.

Wind Affecting the Rectum

Symptoms: dry stool or diarrhea with gas

Treat by enema of medicinal butter with dan khra (purging croton) or dan rog (castor oil plant).

Wind Affecting the Bladder

Signs and symptoms: swelling or cold sensation in the bladder, scant urine, or incontinence

Treat by massage with oil and herbs that benefit the kidneys such as *gze ma* (puncture vine), *lcam pa* (mallow), *sdig srin* (crab), *sug smel* (green cardamom), *rgya tshwa* (ammonium chloride), etc.

Wind Affecting the Uterus

Signs and symptoms: sensation of tightness in the uterus, amenorrhea, or excessive uterine bleeding

Treatment: bone soup, keeping the body warm (especially the lumbar area) and herbal formulas based of *sug smel* (green cardamom)

Wind Affecting the Head

Symptoms: dizziness, mental instability

Treat by massage over the head followed by moxibustion.

Wind Affecting the Ears

Symptoms: hollow sensation, buzzing or ringing in the ears

Treat by fomentation followed by warm ghee poured into the ears.

Wind Affecting the Eyes

Signs and symptoms: red, painful eyes with a bulging feeling

This is treated by applying ghee to the eyelids. The eyes should not be exposed to cold wind.

Wind Affecting the Nose

Signs and symptoms: blocked or runny nose, loss of the sense of smell

This is treated by applying ghee to the nose.

Wind Affecting the Teeth

Signs and symptoms: pain in the teeth, swollen gums

- This is treated by fomentation and moxibustion at the appropriate points.
- A preparation of the four essences—meat, butter, *bu ram* (raw cane sugar) and alcohol—should also be given.

Wind Affecting All the Sense Organs

Signs and symptoms: disturbances in the sense perceptions, such as poor vision, tinnitus, loss of the sense of taste, etc.

This condition is treated with medicinal butter made with *a ru ra* (chebulic myrobalan), *ba ru ra* (beleric myrobalan), and *skyu ru ra* (amla).

Wind Affecting the Entire Body

Signs and symptoms: general symptoms of wind disorders

Any of the modalities available for the general treatment of wind conditions is applicable.

Classification and Treatment by Subdivision of Wind

Disorder of the Life-sustaining Wind

Causative factors: eating rough foods, fasting, strenuous exercise, speaking, thinking or worrying a lot, forcible retention or expulsion of feces or urine

Signs and symptoms: dizziness, emotional instability, difficulty breathing or swallowing
Treatment: massage with sesame oil, and mild inhalation therapy.

Disorder of the Ascending Wind

Causative factors: forcible retention of belching or vomitus, depression or melancholy, physical exertion

Signs and symptoms: impaired speech, fatigue, facial paralysis, loss of mental clarity
Treatment: inhalation, medicinal butter, bone soup, and moxibustion.

Disorder of the Pervasive Wind

Causative factors: incessant travel, hyperactivity, eating rough foods in excess, shock, and fright

Signs and symptoms: restlessness, fainting, mental confusion, talkativeness, anxiety, catatonia
Treatment: *dzA ti* (nutmeg), *snying zho sha* (lapsi tree), medicinal butter made with bone soup, and alcohol made with *bu ram* (raw cane sugar), dried meat, and other warming ingredients

Disorder of the Fire-like Wind

Causative factors: eating hard-to-digest foods, sleeping during the day

Signs and symptoms: anorexia, vomiting, indigestion, blood in the stool

Treatment: fomentation therapy; the powder of *shing kun* (asafetida), *sman sga* (ginger), and *kha ru tshwa* (black salt); moxibustion

Disorder of the Purgative Wind

Causative factors: forcible retention or expulsion of feces, urine, sperm, or gas

Signs and symptoms: pain in the hip bones, bad breath, loose joints, constipation

Treatment: enema, massage, and fomentation therapies; nutritious food that is easy to digest; moxibustion

Wind Combined with Other Humors

Wind and Bile Combined Disorders

Signs and symptoms: fever; yellow eyes, skin, and urine

Treatment: purgation (described in the chapter on bile) followed by cool nourishing foods

Wind and Phlegm Combined Disorders

Signs and symptoms: sensation of cold, heaviness, and mental clouding

Treatment: emesis (described in the chapter on phlegm) followed by light warming foods

If wind and phlegm combine to cause diseases of the heart and sides of the chest, the following two decoctions can be helpful:

- *g.yer ma* (Sichuan pepper), *a ru ra* (chebulic myrobalan), *shing kun* (asafetida), *rgyam tshwa* (rock salt), *shing tsha* (cinnamon), *kha ru tshwa* (black salt), and *ma nu pa tra* (elecampane) together with barley and honey
- *shing kun* (asafetida), *sman sga* (ginger), *se 'bru* (pomegranate), *kha ru tshwa* (black salt), and *ru rta* (costus)

Disorders Caused by Bile

This chapter is derived from the third chapter of the Oral Instruction Tantra and related sources. According to the Buddhist view, there are three fundamental mental afflictions: passion or desire, anger or hatred, and ignorance or delusion. Those three afflictions or poisons are said to arise from basic ignorance of the true nature of reality. Of the three mental poisons, anger or hatred is the fundamental cause of bile disease.

Immediate Causes

Bile is sharp and hot by nature, therefore similar conditions cause it to arise: excessive intake of pungent, sour, salty, or unwholesome foods, or of alcohol, meat, or fat; indigestion; anger; pollution; provocations of energy (i.e. those traditionally said to be caused by evil spirits or sorcery); staying in the sun or other exposure to heat; strenuous activity; and physical injury to vital organs. When those causes meet with other factors, such as the season or bodily constitution, which are also causative of bile conditions, bile conditions arise.

General Diagnosis of Bile Disorders

The general signs and symptoms of bile disorders are:

- Pulse: thin, tight, and with a rapid beat
- Urine: intense yellow color with a strong smell and small bubbles that disappear quickly
- Tongue: covered with a thick yellow coat
- Eyes: yellow or red sclera, cataract
- Jaundice
- Fever
- Insomnia
- Itching
- Fixed pain anywhere in the body, especially in the head, at the nape of the neck, or around the eyes
- Bitter taste or salty mucus in the mouth, nausea, thirst, and vomiting of bilious fluid
- Apathy, discomfort when exposed to heat, and sensations of heat in the body

Diagnosis sometimes needs to be clarified by exploratory treatment or by investigating ameliorating and aggravating factors. If the intake of yogurt, buttermilk, water, or any heavy, cool, or lean food or drink improves the patient's condition, or if the patient's condition improves after undergoing a generic treatment of bile disorders (see below), then a bile condition is indicated. Likewise, if the patient is made worse by eating warm, rich foods such as meat, butter, alcohol, or any other pungent, sour, or oily foods, etc., then this also suggests a bile disorder.

Although bile is hot by nature, there exist hot and cold subtypes of bile disease. The general treatment of bile disorders is therefore divided into two corresponding categories. The differential diagnosis and treatment of each type are described next.

General Treatment of Hot Bile Disorders

When the blood is affected alone or along with the bile, the disorder is of a hot nature. Signs and symptoms are: excessive thirst, tight pulse, urine with a lot of vapor and sediment, bitter taste in the mouth, fever, lack of sleep, yellowish stools, and worsening of the condition when eating rich foods.

Lifestyle and Diet

The patient should be advised to avoid exposure to the sun or other sources of heat, strenuous physical activity, and not to indulge feelings of envy. The surroundings should be cool and pleasant, and the lifestyle should be leisurely. Taking frequent baths, rinsing the head, and wearing new or clean clothes should be encouraged.

The following food and drink are recommended: fresh meat of beef or deer, fresh butter, fresh fruits and vegetables, rice, barley, cold water, yogurt, buttermilk, tea, and any other food or drink that is of cooling nature and easy to digest.

Internal Therapy

Treatment consists of a decoction followed by a powder. The decoction is taken cold and the powder with cold water.

- Decoction: *tig ta* (chiretta), *gser gyi me tog* (bolenggua), *kyi lce* (broad-leaf gentian), *ba sha ka* (Malabar nut tree), and *bong nga dkar po* (white aconite). If there is loss of appetite, ingredients that stimulate digestion can be added, such as *pi pi ling* (long pepper), etc.
- Powder: *gser gyi me tog* (bolenggua), *tig ta* (chiretta)—three parts, or use one part each of *rgya tig* (Indian chiretta), *bal tig* (Nepalese chiretta), and *bod tig*

(Tibetan chiretta); *bong nga dkar po* (white aconite), *ru rta* (costus), *par pa ta* (fumitory), *rtsa mkhris* (rabbit milkweed), *hong len* (picrorhiza grass), *skyer pa'i bar shun* (barberry root middle bark), and *ka ra* (white rock sugar).

External Therapy

Bloodletting is especially indicated for hot bile disorders. Refer to the appropriate chapter for a detailed description of treatment methods.

General Treatment of Cold Bile Disorders

When the bile invades the digestive system or the location of the wind or phlegm humor, the result is a cold-bile disorder. Signs and symptoms are: slow digestion (because of diminished digestive heat), discolored stools, and other signs of cold.

Lifestyle and Diet

The patient should avoid exposure to humidity and strong or cold wind. Recommended foods are fresh butter, fresh mutton, fresh fish, and preserved or dried meat. Food should generally be pungent and include garlic and fresh light foods.

Internal Therapy

The main treatment is a powder made with *se 'bru* (pomegranate), *shing tsha* (cinnamon), *skyu ru ra* (amla), *nim pa* (neem tree), *star bu* (sea buckthorn), *gar nag* (calcined wild-boar stool), and *ka ra* (white rock sugar).

External Therapy

If the therapies mentioned above fail, moxibustion should be performed on the appropriate points. Depending on the patient's condition, sudorific therapy either is contraindicated or should be performed cautiously and for a short time.

Classification and Treatment by Type of Illness

Bile disorders can be classified into four broad categories:

- Bile that increases in its natural location: this is the basic cause of the different classes of fever, which will be presented in subsequent chapters.
- Bile that invades another area: the bile humor can disturb the wind humor, the digestive system, the phlegm humor, or the blood.
- Bile that has lodged itself in the hollow organs, especially the stomach, the liver, or the gallbladder

- Bile that spread throughout the body: this typically represents infectious diseases and may lead to jaundice *(mig ser)* or "yellowing of the muscles" *(sha ser)*. Of those two conditions, the least serious is jaundice, which consists of a slight yellowing of the sclera of the eyes and/or of the skin. When the more serious yellowing of the muscles is present, the entire body is invaded by bile, and a strong yellow discoloration is seen throughout.

Bile Invading the Location of the Wind Humor

Signs and symptoms: flatulence, dry stools, yawning, relief after digesting warm nutritious foods
- The patient should be given mutton, fresh butter, new wine, and warming nutritious food.
- The powder made of *se 'bru* (pomegranate), *pi pi ling* (long pepper), *tig ta* (chiretta), *shing kun* (asafetida), *sman sga* (ginger), *kha ru tshwa* (black salt), *a ru ra* (chebulic myrobalan), and *bu ram* (raw cane sugar) should be given with warm water.
- Medicated enema with butter is very effective.
- Moxibustion is indicated.

Bile Causing Indigestion or Invading the Location of the Phlegm Humor

Signs and symptoms: sensation of heaviness, excessive sleep, nausea, prostration, anxiety, whitish stools

- The patient should be given the powder of *se 'bru* (pomegranate), *shing tsha* (cinnamon), *sug smel* (green cardamom), and *sga skya* (galangal) in order to stimulate the digestive fire.
- Afterward, appropriate emetic and/or purgation therapies (both described in the chapter on phlegm) should be performed.
- Any residual bile should be treated with the decoction of *tig ta* (chiretta), *gser gyi me tog* (bolenggua), and *rgyam tshwa* (rock salt).
- Moxibustion is indicated.

Bile Invading the Location of the Blood

Signs and symptoms: small, dry, pink, or black stools.

- This condition leads to a dark phlegm disorder. It should be treated in the same manner as dark phlegm. Refer to the appropriate chapter for details on the treatment of dark phlegm.

- Moxibustion should then be performed. When the bile has been gathered and brought down to be evacuated through the small intestine (i.e. by means of purgation), the treatment cannot fail.
- If this condition is associated with enlargement of the liver, the following should be given: *cu gang* (bamboo pith), *gur gum* (safflower), *li shi* (clove), *brag zhun* (mineral pitch), *tig ta* (chiretta), *pi pi ling* (long pepper), *a ru ra* (chebulic myrobalan), and *mtshal* (cinnabar). Then strong bloodletting should be performed, followed by the appropriate purgation and moxibustion therapies.

Tumor or Enlargement of the Liver Pressing on the Gallbladder

Signs and symptoms: hardness in the area of the liver and other symptoms of bile- or liver-related illness

- A pill should be made of the following ingredients in calcined form: *'gron thal* (calcined cowrie shell), *mda' rgyus* (precatory bean), *shu dag* (sweet flag), *spyang tsher* (thistle), and *rgyam tshwa* (rock salt).
- Then a small amount of blood should be drawn from the appropriate points.
- Finally moxibustion should be performed.

Bile Causing a Tumor (Gallstones)

Signs and symptoms: loss of strength, jaundice, itching, lack of appetite

- This condition should be treated by purgation and bloodletting. First the patient should be given *gar nag* (calcined wild-boar stool) mixed with *ka ra* (white rock sugar), *se 'bru* (pomegranate), *shing tsha* (cinnamon), *sug smel* (green cardamom), *pi pi ling* (long pepper), and *sga skya* (galangal).
- Then at the appropriate time, the patient should be given *tig ta* (chiretta), *gser gyi me tog* (bolenggua), *bong nga dkar po* (white aconite), *ru rta* (costus), *rtsa mkhris* (rabbit milkweed), *hong len* (picrorhiza grass), *par pa ta* (fumitory), and *skyer pa'i bar shun* (barberry root middle bark).
- Bloodletting should be performed with moderation.
- Moxibustion is indicated.

Even if the disease appears cured, it may persist unseen, and if the condition is left untreated, the patient's accomplishing bile may be weakened.

Bile Causing Jaundice *(mig ser)*

Signs and symptoms: cataract, yellow nails, perspiration, prostration, internal sensation of heat, pain in the eyes and in the bones, poor appetite, thirst, desire to vomit, green- or pink-tinged vision

- The patient should first take a decoction of *tig ta* (chiretta) served cold.
- Then another decoction should be made with *a ru ra* (chebulic myrobalan), *ba ru ra* (beleric myrobalan), *skyu ru ra* (amla), *dur byid* (spurge), *dong ga* (golden shower tree), *lcum rtsa* (rhubarb), *kyi lce* (broad-leaf gentian), *rgun 'brum* (raisin), *hong len* (picrorhiza grass), *bong nga dkar po* (white aconite), and *sle tres* (moonseed).
- This should be followed by bloodletting.

Bile Causing Yellowing of the Muscles *(sha ser)*

Signs and symptoms: loss of strength, insomnia, sensation of heaviness, a milky taste in the mouth, golden coloration of the muscles, white- or yellow-tinged vision, alleviation in the morning or upon eating cooling foods, aggravation around noon

- The following decoction is indicated: *tig ta* (chiretta), *dug mo nyung* (kurchi), *gser gyi me tog* (bolenggua), *hong len* (picrorhiza grass), *ba sha ka* (Malabar nut tree), *bong nga dkar po* (white aconite), and *ba le ka* (birthwort).
- Bloodletting should be performed.
- For purgation, the patient should be given a powder made with *tig ta* (chiretta), *dug mo nyung* (kurchi), *kyi lce* (broad-leaf gentian), and *dur byid* (spurge).
- Then the patient should be given *gur gum* (safflower), *cu gang* (bamboo pith), *gi waM* (elephant or ox gallstone), *ut pal* (Himalayan poppy), *ba sha ka* (Malabar nut tree), *pri yang ku* (nodding dragonhead), and *brag zhun* (mineral pitch). This can be taken with yogurt.

Bile Spread to All the Muscles and Bones

Signs and symptoms are grayish or dark skin, itching, loss of hair and eyebrows, weakness, emaciation, black or spotted fingernails. This condition is the result of not treating either of the above two conditions (jaundice or yellowing of the muscles) for a very long time. It is considered fatal.

Miscellaneous Bile Conditions

Several bile conditions are described in the Oral Instruction Tantra without specific treatment:

- Upward movement of stomach acid
- Bile out of its normal location

- Bad taste in the mouth or excessive salivation
- Downward movement of stomach acid (symptom: hot diarrhea)
- Bile pressed by the growth of the stomach (symptom: excessive hunger or thirst)
- Incoherent speech
- Bile lodged in the hollow organs
- Bile obstructing the channels, causing yellowing of the muscles *(sha ser)* or jaundice *(mig ser)*, mostly because of improper diet

Classification and Treatment by Location

The location of a bile condition progresses along with the severity of the illness. Thus the bile at first is located in the skin, increases in the muscles, then moves in the channels. The bile further gets attached to the bones and falls into the solid organs, to be dispersed through the hollow organs (stomach, intestines, bladder, and uterus). Ultimately, it flowers in the five sense organs (head, eyes, ears, nose, and tongue).

Bile in the Muscles, in the Skin, or Causing a Bad Taste in the Mouth

Long-standing, untreated bile conditions can lead to the spreading of the bile throughout the body. This kind of condition can be very serious or even fatal.

- Signs and symptoms of bile affecting the muscles: dermatitis, pimples, itching, exudation of blood or yellow fluid through the skin
- Symptoms of bile affecting the skin: stickiness of the skin or itching

Treatment for the above is as follows:

- *rgya spos* (clover), *spang spos* (muskroot), *brag spos* (a kind of fern), *a ru ra* (chebulic myrobalan), *shug pa tsher* can (juniper), *lca ba* (angelica), *tang kun nag po* (Wallich milk parsley), *ba lu* (rhododendron), *shu dag* (sweet flag), and *ru rta* (costus) mixed with cow urine, internally or externally. (If cow urine is to be taken internally, it should undergo a process of purification.)
- A paste made of yogurt mixed with *sngon bu* (trailing bellflower) and *srub ka* (*Anemone rivularis*) should be rubbed on the body of the patient.
- Another external preparation can be made with milk cream mixed with *sgog skya* (garlic) and *rgyam tshwa* (rock salt) applied to the patient's body. The patient should then lie in the sun until the paste is dry, and then the residue is scraped off the skin. This treatment should be repeated many times.

Bile Affecting the Channels and Blood Vessels

Signs and symptoms: hot, soft, and itching patches at the joints and muscles that can spread to the entire body, yellowing of the eyes and skin, and bloodletting treatment that yields yellow fluid rather than blood

- The patient should be given a decoction made with two parts of *tig ta* (chiretta) and one part each of *dug mo nyung* (kurchi), *ba le ka* (birthwort), *ba sha ka* (Malabar nut tree), *kyi lce* (broad-leaf gentian), *gser gyi me tog* (bolenggua), and *'om bu* (German tamarisk).
- Vigorous bloodletting should be performed.
- The powder of *ga bur 25* (Camphor 25) may also be given.

Bile Affecting the Bones

Signs and symptoms: pain in the joints, pustules, and atrophy and swelling of the joints

- Prolonged purgation therapy should be administered, using *tig ta* (chiretta)—three parts, or use one part each of *rgya tig* (Indian chiretta), *bal tig* (Nepalese chiretta), and *bod tig* (Tibetan chiretta); *a ru ra* (chebulic myrobalan), *ba ru ra* (beleric myrobalan), *skyu ru ra* (amla), *khron bu* (Euphorbia stracheyi), *lcum rtsa* (rhubarb), and *stab seng* (Korean ash).
- The formula *ga bur 25* (Camphor 25) may also be given.
- Cooling foods and baths are recommended.

Bile Affecting the Muscles, Blood, and Ligaments

The herbs *ga bur* (camphor), *tsan dan dkar po* (white sandalwood), *tsan dan dmar po* (red sandalwood), the "three *ge sar*" (one part each of the three different parts of the silk cotton tree flower), and *ut pal* (Himalayan poppy) should be made into a syrup with butter, *ka ra* (white rock sugar), and *sbrang rtsi* (honey) and taken orally.

Bile Affecting the Solid Organs

When the hollow organs are affected by bile, the following formula is to be used and modified appropriately: *tig ta* (chiretta)—three parts, or use one part each of *rgya tig* (Indian chiretta), *bal tig* (Nepalese chiretta), and *bod tig* (Tibetan chiretta); *gser gyi me tog* (bolenggua), *dug mo nyung* (kurchi), *rgun 'brum* (raisin), *kyi lce* (broad-leaf gentian), and *bong nga dkar po* (white aconite). Modify the formula based on the organ affected as follows:

- Bile affecting the heart: chest discomfort, yellow tongue, insomnia, and desire for cooling foods and drinks. Add *dzA ti* (nutmeg).
- Bile affecting the lungs: yellowish mucus. Add *shing mngar* (licorice), *cu gang* (bamboo pith), and a *krong* (sandwort).
- Bile affecting the liver: brown discoloration of the muscles *(sha ser)*, pain above the liver, headache, burning sensation in the eyes, and thick saliva. Add *brag zhun* (mineral pitch), *gur gum* (safflower), and *ba sha ka* (Malabar nut tree).
- Bile affecting the spleen: reddish moist tongue, diarrhea, gas, swelling of the left leg, and pain in the bones and joints. Add *ru rta* (costus), *se 'bru* (pomegranate), and *pi pi ling* (long pepper).
- Bile affecting the kidneys: heaviness of the legs, sneezing, lumbar pain, and yellow discoloration at the back of the ears. Add *shug pa tsher* can (juniper), *sug smel* (green cardamom), *btsod* (Indian madder), *'bri mog* (Tibetan groomwell), and *rgya skyegs* (shellac).

Bile Affecting the Hollow Organs

- Bile affecting the stomach: diarrhea and vomiting with bilious fluid
- Bile affecting the intestines: diarrhea with bilious fluid
- Bile affecting the bladder: salivation, difficult urination, oliguria, or frequent urination
- Bile affecting the uterus: yellowish vaginal discharge

In all the above cases, the appropriate purgation therapy should be performed.

Bile Affecting the Head

Signs and symptoms are pain in the head and at the sutures of the skull, aggravated by exposure to the sun, by yogurt intake, and in the fall. Purgation, emesis (described in the chapter on phlegm), and bloodletting should be performed as well as the therapies below:

- A powder made of *tig ta* (chiretta), *gser gyi me tog* (bolenggua), *bong nga dkar po* (white aconite), *ru rta* (costus), *par pa ta* (fumitory), *hong len* (picrorhiza grass), *rtsa mkhris* (rabbit milkweed), and *skyer pa'i bar shun* (barberry root middle bark) should be mixed in water and applied to the head.
- Moxibustion is indicated.
- Medicinal butter made with *a ru ra* (chebulic myrobalan), *ba ru ra* (beleric myrobalan), and *skyu ru ra* (amla) may be beneficial.

Bile Affecting the Eyes

Signs and symptoms: yellow sclera, burning sensation in the eyes, tears

Treatment for this condition is bloodletting followed by external application of concentrated extract of *skyer pa* (barberry).

Bile Affecting the Ears

Signs and symptoms: severe pain and burning sensation in the ears, discharge from the ears

A decoction of *ru rta* (costus), *sran ma gyi me tog* (legume flower), *gser gyi me tog* (bolenggua), *a ru ra* (chebulic myrobalan), and *ba ru ra* (beleric myrobalan) should be thoroughly filtered and then poured into the ear.

Bile Affecting the Nose

Signs and symptoms: yellow mucus in the nose

The inside of the nose should be rinsed with salt water. Then a paste of *gur gum* (safflower) mixed with warm ghee should be applied on the nose.

Bile Affecting the Tongue

Signs and symptoms: yellow tongue, different kinds of tastes in the mouth

The blood vessels under the tongue should be bled, and then the patient should be given some sweet drugs made into a paste to keep in the mouth.

Jaundice

Signs and symptoms are the same as yellowing of the muscles *(sha ser)* or jaundice *(mig ser)*. A number of treatments are suggested below:

- Cold decoction of *tig ta* (chiretta)
- *a ru ra* (chebulic myrobalan), *ba ru ra* (beleric myrobalan), *skyu ru ra* (amla), *dur byid* (spurge), *dong ga* (golden shower tree), *lcum rtsa* (rhubarb), *kyi lce* (broad-leaf gentian), *rgun 'brum* (raisin), *hong len* (picrorhiza grass), *bong nga dkar po* (white aconite), and *sle tres* (moonseed). This formula is said to relieve heat from the abdomen.
- Bloodletting should be performed at the appropriate points.
- *sle tres* (moonseed), *tig ta* (chiretta), *sman sga* (ginger), *sgog skya* (garlic), *a ru ra* (chebulic myrobalan), *hong len* (picrorhiza grass), *dug mo nyung* (kurchi), and *ka ra* (white rock sugar)

- *ga bur* (camphor), *cu gang* (bamboo pith), *gur gum* (safflower), *tsan dan dkar po* (white sandalwood), *ba sha ka* (Malabar nut tree), *hong len* (picrorhiza grass), *pad ma ge sar* (silk cotton tree), and *ka ra* (white rock sugar)

Classification and Treatment by Subdivision of Bile

Disorder of the Digestive Bile

Symptoms and signs: yellow coating on the tongue, thirst, indigestion, poor appetite

For treatment, give the patient a decoction of *rgya tshwa* (ammonium chloride), *rgyam tshwa* (rock salt), and *kha ru tshwa* (black salt), followed by emetic therapy based on *gser gyi phud bu* (sponge gourd).

Disorder of the Color-Transforming Bile

Symptoms and signs: jaundice, fullness of the stomach, sensation of heaviness, lack of strength

Treatment: purgation therapy; the patient should then be given a powder of *'jam 'bras* (Indian beech) with *tig ta* (chiretta). Then bloodletting should be performed on the bile channels.

Disorder of the Accomplishing Bile

Symptoms and signs: palpitations, difficulty breathing, thirst, nausea, shivering, burning sensation in the chest

- The following powder should be given: *a ga ru* (eaglewood), *dzA ti* (nutmeg), *gur gum* (safflower), *a ru ra* (chebulic myrobalan), *tig ta* (chiretta), *nA ga ge sar* (silk cotton tree), with six parts of *ka ra* (white rock sugar).
- Gentle massage should be done on the upper part of the body, followed by bloodletting.

Disorder of the Vision-Producing Bile

Symptoms and signs: headache, especially after drinking alcohol; myopia

- The patient should be given a paste made with *tig ta* (chiretta), *gser gyi me tog* (bolenggua), *bong nga dkar po* (white aconite), *ma nu pa tra* (elecampane), *pi pi ling* (long pepper), *ba le ka* (birthwort), and *sbrang rtsi* (honey).
- Cold water should be applied over the eyes.

Disorder of the Complexion-Clearing Bile

Symptoms and signs: sensation of heat in the muscles and skin, dark skin discoloration

- Apply a paste made with *tsan dan dkar po* (white sandalwood) and *gur gum* (safflower).
- Perform bloodletting over the capillaries.

Bile Combined with Other Humors

When a disorder is the result of a combination of bile with another humor, the signs and symptoms that pertain to that humor will be present along with those of bile conditions, and the other humors should be treated in the appropriate manner.

For combined wind and bile disorders accompanied with depletion of the seven bodily constituents, medicinal butter made with the following ingredients is particularly effective: *tig ta* (chiretta), *hong len* (picrorhiza grass), *ba sha ka* (Malabar nut tree), *sbrang rtsi* (honey), and *kyi lce* (broad-leaf gentian). This medicinal butter is to be mixed with the powder of *gur gum* (safflower) and the "three *ge sar*" (one part each of the three different parts of the silk cotton tree flower).

Treatment of Persistent or Residual Bile Disorder

If the patient is strong, the powder of *gi waM* (elephant or ox gallstone) and other kinds of bile, three parts in total, along with one part each of *gur gum* (safflower) and *ka ra* (white rock sugar) should be taken with milk. Then the patient should be given *stab seng* (Korean ash), *gser gyi me tog* (bolenggua), and *ka ra* (white rock sugar) mixed with milk.

If the patient's bodily constituents are depleted and the wind humor is disturbed, medicinal butter made with *tig ta* (chiretta) should be given.

The patient should be attentive to observe the appropriate diet and lifestyle recommendations for up to a year.

DISORDERS CAUSED BY PHLEGM

This chapter is derived from the fourth chapter of the Oral Instruction Tantra and related sources. According to the Buddhist view, there are three fundamental mental afflictions: passion or desire, anger or hatred, and ignorance or delusion. Those three afflictions or poisons are said to arise from basic ignorance of the true nature of reality. Of the three mental poisons, delusion is the fundamental cause of phlegm disease.

Phlegm is cold, heavy, and dull by nature. Because of that, it is said to be the cause of all internal (organ) diseases, starting with the reduction of the power of digestion. Impairment of the power of digestion *(ma zhu)* is a related condition described in the sixth chapter of the Oral Instruction Tantra. This is a chronic condition caused by phlegm and usually combined with other humors. This condition is treated in a later chapter of the Oral Instruction Tantra because it is more specific than a general phlegm condition.

Immediate Causes

The causes of phlegm disorders include a diet excessive in bitter or sweet foods or in foods with heavy, cold, or greasy qualities. This includes raw cereals or pulses, animal fats, vegetable oils, sugar, radish, cottonseed, raw or under-cooked foods, slightly burned foods, dairy products, or drinking cold water or cold tea to excess. Overeating, eating a meal before the previous meal was digested, inactivity, sleeping during the day, and chronic exposure to humidity are other possible causes of phlegm disorders.

General Diagnosis of Phlegm Disorders

The general signs and symptoms of phlegm disorders are:

- Pulse: weak, slow, sunken, and almost imperceptible
- Urine: whitish and turbid with tiny bubbles and little smell or fume
- Tongue: covered with a pale-white moist coat
- A sticky sensation in the mouth with a reduced ability to taste foods
- Pale face, eyes, tongue, and gums, and swollen eyelids
- Abundant saliva and mucus
- Dull-mindedness, sensation of heaviness, sleepiness, apathy, procrastination, or laziness

- Lack of appetite, nausea, poor digestion, stomach discomfort, vomiting and diarrhea with undigested food or mucus in the stools
- Lumbar discomfort or pain, itching, slackening or thickening of the skin, and loose or enlarged joints
- Swelling of the neck[8]
- Viscous, light-colored blood revealed by bloodletting

The above symptoms are aggravated in the spring, in rainy weather, in the morning, in late afternoon, and immediately after eating.

A diagnosis of phlegm disorder can be further confirmed by ameliorating and aggravating conditions. If the condition improves after eating lamb, beef, honey, grains grown in dry areas, or pungent, sour, or astringent foods, or foods with rough, warm, and sharp qualities, or when staying in warm places, or after physical exercise, then the diagnosis of phlegm can be confirmed. Likewise, the following aggravating factors can help confirm the diagnosis of phlegm: hard-to-digest meat, withered greens, stale foods, foods left to dry after cooking, sweet or bitter foods or foods with heavy, cold, or blunt qualities, overeating, or sleeping during the day.

General Treatment of Phlegm Disorders

Since phlegm is very cold by nature, the general treatment of phlegm is warming. In general, phlegm affects the stomach and the digestive process. Therefore treatment of the stomach is important in the treatment of phlegm.

The rest of this section describes the main modalities used to treat phlegm in general. According to the Oral Instruction Tantra, if those general measures do not bring improvement, then it is better to refrain from those and wait.

Lifestyle and Diet

The patient should eat dry ripe grain and other kinds of warm, light, and rough foods and drinks. Alcohol is advisable in moderate amounts. Hot water, water boiled with ginger, mutton, beef, and fish are recommended. The patient should refrain from overeating, and from any foods that aggravate phlegm (sweet, cold, oily foods, etc.).

The patient should keep the body well covered, stay in warm sunny places, exercise the body and the voice, not oversleep, and in general refrain from activities that cause the phlegm humor to arise.

[8.] This may be enlargement of the thyroid.

Internal Therapy

The following decoctions are recommended for the general treatment of phlegm:

- *rgyam tshwa* (rock salt), *bca' sga* (fresh ginger), and *a ru ra* (chebulic myrobalan)
- The above plus *pi pi ling* (long pepper)
- *rgyam tshwa* (rock salt), *bre ga* (pennycress) and *pi pi ling* (long pepper)
- *pi pi ling* (long pepper), *na le sham* (black pepper), and *sman sga* (ginger)

The following powders are recommended for the general treatment of phlegm, especially phlegm that affects the upper part of the body:

- *se 'bru* (pomegranate), *shing tsha* (cinnamon), *sug smel* (green cardamom), and *sga skya* (galangal)
- Especially for recent or chronic indigestion: *se 'bru* (pomegranate), *shing tsha* (cinnamon), *sug smel* (green cardamom), *pi pi ling* (long pepper), *rgyam tshwa* (rock salt), *kha ru tshwa* (black salt), *na le sham* (black pepper), and *bca' sga* (fresh ginger)
- *dwa lis* (rhododendron), *shing tsha* (cinnamon), *sug smel* (green cardamom), *ka ko la* (black cardamom), *zi ra nag po* (fennelflower), *pi pi ling* (long pepper), and *na le sham* (black pepper)
- *'jam 'bras* (fever nut) alone
- *pi pi ling* (long pepper), *na le sham* (black pepper), *sman sga* (ginger), *dbyi mong* (clematis), and *tsi tra ka* (wild leadwort)
- *kha ru tshwa* (black salt) alone
- This powder is useful to stimulate the appetite and improve digestion. It also alleviates belching and colic: *se 'bru* (pomegranate), *shing tsha* (cinnamon), *sug smel* (green cardamom), *sga skya* (galangal), *zi ra nag po* (fennelflower), *kha ru tshwa* (black salt), and *sman sga* (ginger).

External Therapy

If cold is severe, moxibustion is beneficial.

Emesis or Purgation

If there is residual phlegm, emesis or purgation should be resorted according to the location of the phlegm. For phlegm in the upper part of the body, emesis is indicated. If the phlegm resides in the intestines, purgation is appropriate. The effect of purgation or emesis does not depend on the choice of herb alone but also on the season of harvest: herbs picked in the spring tend to be emetic, while those picked in the fall will tend to be purgative. Examples of herbs used for emesis and / or purgation include *thar nu* (Wallich spurge) and *dur byid* (spurge).

Classification and Treatment by Type of Illness

Phlegm disorders can be classified into six broad categories as described in this section.

Phlegm in the Upper Part of the Stomach

Signs and symptoms: nausea, difficult digestion, pain on eating relieved after digestion

Treat by giving a decoction of *pi pi ling* (long pepper), *na le sham* (black pepper), *sman sga* (ginger), *rgyam tshwa* (rock salt), and *kha ru tshwa* (black salt).

Phlegm in the Whole Stomach

Signs and symptoms: belching, abdominal swelling, slow digestion, nausea, emaciation, constipation, chest discomfort, vomiting with mucus or undigested foods

This disorder is treated by administering calcined *cong zhi* (calcite) and other sharp substances. This should be followed up with purgation or emesis and finally by giving formulas based on *se 'bru* (pomegranate). If the patient does not get better, moxibustion should be performed.

Phlegm Affecting the Fire-like Wind

This condition is caused by the ingestion of cold or raw foods and exposure to cold weather or cold water. Excessive purgation or bloodletting also weakens the digestive bile and the fire-like wind, thus making the condition worse.

Signs and symptoms are sensation of cold alleviated by warming diet or activity, indigestion, poor appetite, feeling of fullness even with an empty stomach, flatulence, belching, diarrhea with undigested food in the stools, weakness, and emaciation. If there is fever, the signs and symptoms of fever remain hidden. The following formulas can be helpful:

- The powder of *'jam 'bras* (fever nut) alone or *se 'bru* (pomegranate) alone
- *pi pi ling* (long pepper), *na le sham* (black pepper), *sman sga* (ginger), *dbyi mong* (clematis), and *tsi tra ka* (wild leadwort)
- *dzA ti* (nutmeg), *sug smel* (green cardamom), and *ka ko la* (black cardamom)

- *byi tang ga* (false black pepper), *srub ka (Anemone rivularis)*, *'jam 'bras* (fever nut), *rgyam tshwa* (rock salt), *kha ru tshwa* (black salt), and *bu ram* (raw cane sugar)

The above promote the power of digestion and should be given with warm water. Other remedies include:

- One part each of *rgyam tshwa* (rock salt), *la la phud, dbyi mong* (clematis), *pi pi ling* (long pepper), and *sman sga* (ginger) should be mixed with five parts of calcined *a ru ra* (chebulic myrobalan). This remedy is said to be the best to stimulate digestion.
- A suppository can be prepared with ghee mixed with *shing kun* (asafetida), *kha ru tshwa* (black salt), *pi pi ling* (long pepper), *na le sham* (black pepper), *sman sga* (ginger) and *sgog skya* (garlic) to stimulate the power of digestion.
- Moxibustion is indicated.

Phlegm Causing Blockage of the Throat

It is said that when phlegm obstructs the throat, the patient is unable to take food and may die. Signs and symptoms are difficulty swallowing or breathing, emaciation, weakness, and inability to take food or drink. The following formulas can be helpful:

- *pi pi ling* (long pepper), *na le sham* (black pepper), *sman sga* (ginger), *dbyi mong* (clematis), and *tsi tra ka* (wild leadwort)
- *dzA ti* (nutmeg), *sug smel* (green cardamom), *ka ko la* (black cardamom), and *li shi* (clove)
- *shing kun* (asafetida), *byi tang ga* (false black pepper), and *rgyam tshwa* (rock salt) ground into a fine powder for snuffing
- The powder of *srub ka (Anemone rivularis)* and *lce tsha* (buttercup) mixed with *sbrang rtsi* (honey)

Afterward, the patient should drink hot water to eliminate residual morbid matter. Emesis or purgation can then be given. Moxibustion is also indicated.

Phlegm of the White Arthritis *(bad kan grum bu dkar po)*

Signs and symptoms are pain around the stomach and liver, indigestion even of adequate foods, diarrhea, vomiting, pain in the calves, muscles, and orbits, stomach reflux, and arthritis of the limbs. The following formulas can be helpful:

- Decoction of *shing kun* (asafetida), *rgya tshwa* (ammonium chloride), and *dbyi mong* (clematis)

- Powder of *sug smel* (green cardamom), *ru rta* (costus), *rgyam tshwa* (rock salt), *pi pi ling* (long pepper), *gla rtsi* (musk), and *byi tang ga* (false black pepper)
- Decoction of *se 'bru* (pomegranate), *pi pi ling* (long pepper), *na le sham* (black pepper), *sman sga* (ginger), *a ru ra* (chebulic myrobalan), *rgyam tshwa* (rock salt), *ma nu pa tra* (elecampane), *'u su* (coriander), *da trig* (schisandra), and *ma ru rtse* (flame of the forest) prepared with *ka ra* (white rock sugar) and *sbrang rtsi* (honey)

The patient should stay in a warm and dry area.

Phlegm Causing Indigestion

This condition is said to be caused by parasites. Signs and symptoms are hunger even after eating, weakness and emaciation even with an adequate diet, and trembling of the legs or knees.

- The patient should take *bca' sga* (fresh ginger), *kha ru tshwa* (black salt), *a ru ra* (chebulic myrobalan), and *skyu ru ra* (amla) along with *ka ra* (white rock sugar).
- Emesis should be performed repeatedly, followed by moxibustion.

Classification and Treatment by Location

The location of a phlegm condition progresses along with the severity of the illness. Thus the phlegm at first causes stickiness of the skin, grows in the muscles, produces stiffness of the channels, attaches itself to the bones, falls upon the solid organs, gets submerged in the hollow organs, and finally "blossoms" in the sense organs (head, eyes, eyes, ears, nose, and tongue).

Phlegm Causing Stickiness of the Skin

Signs and symptoms: decrease of body heat, greasy skin

- The powder of *pi pi ling* (long pepper), *na le sham* (black pepper), and *sman sga* (ginger) should be given to the patient with butter.
- Massage and exposure to sunlight are beneficial.

Phlegm Growing in the Muscles

Signs and symptoms: decrease of body heat, swelling or loosening of the flesh, accumulation of grimy material on the skin or discoloration of the skin, lethargy, sensation of heaviness, poor appetite, formation of new moles

- The patient will benefit from mutton or yak-bull noodle soup.
- This powder may be given to the patient: *se 'bru* (pomegranate), *shing tsha* (cinnamon), *sug smel* (green cardamom), *pi pi ling* (long pepper), *rgyam tshwa* (rock salt), *kha ru tshwa* (black salt), *na le sham* (black pepper), and *bca' sga* (fresh ginger).
- Abdominal exercise is recommended.

Phlegm Causing Stiffness of the Channels

Signs and symptoms: cold sensation, stiffness of the body, sensation of heaviness

- Different types of salts should be given to the patient, notably *rgyam tshwa* (rock salt) and *kha ru tshwa* (black salt).
- Fomentation therapy (the application of warm substances on the surface of the body) is recommended.

Phlegm Attached to the Bones

Signs and symptoms: pain and sensation of cold in the bones, swelling, stiffness, or loosening of the joints

- Raw cane sugar alcohol mixed with *pi pi ling* (long pepper), *na le sham* (black pepper), and *sman sga* (ginger) should be given to the patient.
- Massage with butter is indicated.
- Moxibustion on the joints after applying cold mud is indicated.

Phlegm Affecting the Heart

Signs and symptoms: mental dullness, poor appetite, stiffness of the shoulders, sensation of heaviness

- First, emesis therapy should be given.
- Then the patient should be given *se 'bru* (pomegranate), *shing tsha* (cinnamon), *sug smel* (green cardamom), *sga skya* (galangal), *dzA ti* (nutmeg), *shing kun* (asafetida), and *kha ru tshwa* (black salt) with *sbrang rtsi* (honey) and *ka ra* (white rock sugar) in warm water.
- Alternatively, *dzA ti* (nutmeg), *pi pi ling* (long pepper), *na le sham* (black pepper), *sman sga* (ginger), *sug smel* (green cardamom), *zi ra nag po* (fennelflower), and *ka ko la* (black cardamom) may be given with *ka ra* (white rock sugar).
- Moxibustion should complete the course of treatment.

Phlegm Affecting the Lungs

Signs and symptoms: sensation of fullness in the chest, dizziness, loss of appetite, expectoration of dark mucus

- First, emesis therapy should be given.
- Then the patient should be given *se 'bru* (pomegranate), *shing tsha* (cinnamon), *sug smel* (green cardamom), *sga skya* (galangal), *star bu* (sea buckthorn), *ru rta* (costus), and *cu gang* (bamboo pith) with *sbrang rtsi* (honey) and *ka ra* (white rock sugar) in warm water.
- Alternatively, *se 'bru* (pomegranate), *pi pi ling* (long pepper), *na le sham* (black pepper), *sman sga* (ginger), *zi ra dkar po* (cumin), *zi ra nag po* (fennelflower), *shing tsha* (cinnamon), and *sug smel* (green cardamom) may be given with *bu ram* (raw cane sugar).
- Moxibustion should complete the course of treatment.

Phlegm Affecting the Liver

Signs and symptoms are pain in the liver area after eating and vomiting of bluish liquid. This condition may be caused by parasites.

- The patient should be given *pi pi ling* (long pepper), *na le sham* (black pepper), *sman sga* (ginger), *se 'bru* (pomegranate), *shing tsha* (cinnamon), *kha ru tshwa* (black salt), and *gur gum* (safflower) mixed with *ka ra* (white rock sugar).
- Moxibustion is indicated.

Phlegm Affecting the Spleen

Signs and symptoms: lethargy, difficulty breathing, flatulence, belching, diarrhea with stools the same color as the foods previously ingested

- The patient should be given *se 'bru* (pomegranate), *rgyam tshwa* (rock salt), *pi pi ling* (long pepper), *na le sham* (black pepper), *sman sga* (ginger), *thal tshwa* (a type of salt that is hot in taste and warm in power, perhaps equivalent to black salt), *kha ru tshwa* (black salt), and *lce myang tshwa* (a white natural salt with a red hue found in water, sweet in taste, warm in power, and beneficial for the eyes and for digestion without increasing bile) mixed with *bur dkar* (white raw cane sugar).
- Moxibustion is indicated.

Phlegm Affecting the Kidneys

Signs and symptoms: lumbar pain, difficulty passing stools or urine, hearing loss, aggravation of symptoms when exposed to cold or dampness

- The patient should be given *pi pi ling* (long pepper), *na le sham* (black pepper), *sman sga* (ginger), *sug smel* (green cardamom), *rgya tshwa* (ammonium chloride), *lcam pa* (mallow), *sdig srin* (crab), *gser gyis bye ma* (vermiculite), *a ru ra* (chebulic myrobalan), *ba ru ra* (beleric myrobalan), and *skyu ru ra* (amla) along with *bu ram* (raw cane sugar) and alcohol.
- Moxibustion is indicated.

Phlegm Affecting the Stomach

Signs and symptoms: discomfort and heavy sensation in the stomach, heartburn, indigestion

- The powder of *se 'bru* (pomegranate), *shing tsha* (cinnamon), *sug smel* (green cardamom), *pi pi ling* (long pepper), and *sga skya* (galangal) should be given to the patient.
- Alternatively, *kha ru tshwa* (black salt), *da trig* (schisandra), and *shing kun* (asafetida) may be given.
- Moxibustion should be given at the end of the course of herbal treatment.

Phlegm Affecting the Intestines

- Signs and symptoms of phlegm affecting the large intestine: flatulence, pain after eating
- Signs and symptoms of phlegm affecting the small intestine: diarrhea with mucus in the stools, sensation of heaviness
- For either condition, use *shing tsha* (cinnamon), *pi pi ling* (long pepper), *na le sham* (black pepper), *sman sga* (ginger), *dbyi mong* (clematis), *tsi tra ka* (wild leadwort), *byi tang ga* (false black pepper), *shing kun* (asafetida), and *kha ru tshwa* (black salt) taken with *bu ram* (raw cane sugar).
- Moxibustion is indicated.

Phlegm Affecting the Gallbladder

Signs and symptoms: jaundice, indigestion, sensation of heaviness, sleepiness

- The powder of *se 'bru* (pomegranate), *shing tsha* (cinnamon), *sug smel* (green cardamom), and *sga skya* (galangal) may be given.

- This formula may also be used: *rgyam tshwa* (rock salt), *gser gyi me tog* (bolenggua), and *sga skya* (galangal).
- Purgation and moxibustion therapies are indicated.

Phlegm Affecting the Bladder

The main symptom is whitish cloudy urine with a sticky appearance. This condition is associated with diabetes, where the bladder is affected by loss of heat from the kidneys.

The following herbs are to be taken with alcohol: *rgyam tshwa* (rock salt), *pi pi ling* (long pepper), *na le sham* (black pepper), *sman sga* (ginger), *sug smel* (green cardamom), and *lcam pa* (mallow).

Phlegm Affecting the Uterus

Signs and symptoms: sensation of cold in the lower parts of the body, yellow fluid in the menstrual blood

- The patient should be given a powder of *pi pi ling* (long pepper), *na le sham* (black pepper), *sman sga* (ginger), *sug smel* (green cardamom), *a ru ra* (chebulic myrobalan), *'u su* (coriander), *g.yer ma* (Sichuan pepper), *zi ra dkar po* (cumin), *kha ru tshwa* (black salt), *mtsho tshwa* (lake salt), *shing tsha* (cinnamon), *tig ta* (chiretta), and *go snyod* (caraway).
- An ambiguity in the text can be read either as triple the dosage of the above formula or as the "three-dose remedy" mentioned as an alternative: one part of a salt mixture, one part of the Three Pungent Drug mixture, and one part of the Three Fruit mixture. The salt mixture is made of equal amounts of *rgya tshwa* (ammonium chloride), *rgyam tshwa* (rock salt), *lce myang tshwa* (described above in the section "Phlegm Affecting the Spleen"), *kha ru tshwa* (black salt), *rtsab ru tshwa* (crag halite), *rwa tshwa* (salt made from horn), *shing tsha* (cinnamon), *mdze tshwa* (Glauber's salt), *thal tshwa* (described above in the section "Phlegm Affecting the Spleen"), and *bul tog* (soda ash). The Three Pungent Drug mixture and the Three Fruit mixture are described in the chapter on herb compounding. This remedy is especially effective for benign uterine tumors. It is said that on taking this remedy, tumors disappear the way wood burns down to ash.
- Hot fomentation, moxibustion, and a moderate intake of alcohol are recommended.

Phlegm Affecting the Head

Signs and symptoms: sensation of heaviness in the head, lethargy, poor digestion, loss of appetite

The patient should be given emetic therapy based on *ri sho* (leopard plant) followed by the powder of *se 'bru* (pomegranate), *shing tsha* (cinnamon), *sug smel* (green cardamom), *pi pi ling* (long pepper), *rgyam tshwa* (rock salt), *kha ru tshwa* (black salt), *na le sham* (black pepper), and *bca' sga* (fresh ginger).

Phlegm Affecting the Eyes

Signs and symptoms: swelling around the eyes, tearing

The patient should be given a powder made by burning shavings of *ra gan* (brass) to apply on the eyelids, and eat fish.

Phlegm Affecting the Ears

Signs and symptoms: cold sensation and congestion in the ears, hearing loss

The patient should have a well-filtered decoction of *shing kun* (asafetida) and *rgya tshwa* (ammonium chloride) poured into the ears.

Phlegm Affecting the Nose

Signs and symptoms: nasal obstruction, sensation of fullness in the nose

Inhalation therapy based on medicines with sharp power should be given.

Phlegm Affecting the Tongue

Signs and symptoms: stiffness of the tongue, loss of the sense of taste

A gargle should be prepared with pungent drugs and given to the patient.

Classification and Treatment by Subdivision of Phlegm

Disorder of the Supporting Phlegm

Symptoms and signs: poor appetite, sensation of fullness in the chest, acute pain at the chest and back, heartburn, acid reflux, poor digestion

- Emesis therapy should be given.

- The powder of se 'bru (pomegranate), shing tsha (cinnamon), sug smel (green cardamom), pi pi ling (long pepper), and sga skya (galangal) should then be given to the patient.
- Alternatively, this formula can be given with ka ra (white rock sugar): se 'bru (pomegranate), cong zhi (calcite), sug smel (green cardamom), pi pi ling (long pepper), ru rta (costus), and gur gum (safflower).
- Moxibustion is indicated.

Disorder of the Decomposing Phlegm

Symptoms and signs: poor digestion or assimilation of food, belching, hardening of the stomach

- For treatment, se 'bru (pomegranate), rgyam tshwa (rock salt), and sle tres (moonseed) should be given.
- Moxibustion is indicated.

Disorder of the Gustatory Phlegm

Symptoms and signs: lack of taste, absence of thirst, cold sensation in the tongue, pain in the lips, hoarseness, inability to take food manifesting as diarrhea or vomiting

- The decoction of a ru ra (chebulic myrobalan), ba ru ra (beleric myrobalan), and skyu ru ra (amla) is the main treatment.
- The above may also be augmented with star bu (sea buckthorn), bca' sga (fresh ginger), and shing mngar (licorice) taken with sbrang rtsi (honey).
- Moxibustion is indicated.

Disorder of the Satisfying Phlegm

Symptoms and signs: heaviness of the head, blurred vision, hearing loss, sneezing, abundant mucus or saliva, frequent colds, sensation of heaviness at the top of the head

- For treatment, emesis and inhalation therapies are recommended.
- Moxibustion is indicated.

Disorder of the Connective Phlegm

Symptoms and signs: impaired movement; swollen, painful, or dislocated joints
- For treatment, the powder of a ru ra (chebulic myrobalan), gla rtsi (musk), sman sga (ginger), and bong khrag (donkey blood) should be given.

- A paste should be made by mixing ghee with *thal ka rdo rje* (foetid cassia) and applied to the body.
- Moxibustion is indicated.

Phlegm Combined with Other Humors

Phlegm conditions that involve the wind humor or the bile humor will also manifest symptoms that pertain to that humor. Such combined disorders should be treated in ways consistent with the treatment of each humor affected.

Yellow Phlegm

This condition is said to arise from an overflow of bile. Signs and symptoms of a yellow-phlegm condition include:

- A dull pulse that feels empty on pressure
- Yellowish urine
- Stomach discomfort and poor appetite
- Pain in the orbits
- Burning sensation after drinking alcohol
- Burning sensation in the stomach, acid reflux, or bilious vomiting
- Diarrhea when staying in a damp environment or after eating sour or spoiled foods
- Discomfort after eating roasted grain, goat meat, old butter, etc. or after drinking alcohol

When present for a long time, this condition can turn into a dark-phlegm disorder or a bile disorder. Several possible treatments are described below:

- Decoction of *rgyam tshwa* (rock salt), *bca' sga* (fresh ginger), *a ru ra* (chebulic myrobalan), *pi pi ling* (long pepper), *se 'bru* (pomegranate), *shing tsha* (cinnamon), *sug smel* (green cardamom), *pi pi ling* (long pepper), *rgyam tshwa* (rock salt), *kha ru tshwa* (black salt), *na le sham* (black pepper), and *bca' sga* (fresh ginger). (The duplication of ingredients reflects the combinations of two formulas. The dosage of the duplicate ingredients should be repeated.)
- Emesis based on *gser gyi phud bu* (sponge gourd)
- Hot decoction of *ma nu pa tra* (elecampane), *a ru ra* (chebulic myrobalan), *sle tres* (moonseed), *kaNDa ka ri* (two-flowered raspberry), *sman sga* (ginger), *dong ga* (golden shower tree), and *lcum rtsa* (rhubarb)
- *se 'bru* (pomegranate), *cong zhi* (calcite), *sug smel* (green cardamom), *pi pi ling* (long pepper), *ru rta* (costus), and *gur gum* (safflower)

- Fresh meat, milk, and butter should be included in the patient's diet.
- Moxibustion is indicated.

Dark Phlegm

This condition is associated with impurity of the blood. Signs and symptoms of a dark-phlegm condition include:

- Pain in the stomach, in the liver, and around the shoulders
- Diarrhea and/or vomiting of reddish material, belching
- Sensation of heaviness
- Discomfort around the heart
- Constant appetite, even after eating
- Aggravation from anything hot or cold
- Sudden occurrence or disappearance of pain without apparent cause

This formula is representative of a general approach to treatment: *se 'bru* (pomegranate), *bse yab* (Chinese quince), *star bu* (sea buckthorn), *skyu ru ra* (amla), *sga skya* (galangal), *ma nu pa tra* (elecampane), *'u su* (coriander), *ut pal* (Himalayan poppy), and *pi pi ling* (long pepper) taken with *ka ra* (white rock sugar) and warm water. This condition and its treatment are described in further detail in the next chapter.

Disorders Caused by Dark Phlegm

This chapter is derived from the fifth chapter of the Oral Instruction Tantra and related sources. The disease entity known as dark phlegm is said to be the result of the disturbance of all three humors along with that of the blood. In general, internal disorders are caused by dark phlegm. Dark phlegm can thus be considered a prime example of a disease pattern that involves multiple humors and is therefore difficult to cure.

Immediate Causes

Dark phlegm has two possible types of immediate causes: one related to heat and the other related to cold. The hot variety of dark-phlegm disorder is caused by the disturbance of the blood as a result of a heat condition, trauma, or excessive surgical intervention. The heat condition may be the result of the excessive intake of pungent or sour foods. Since the liver stores the blood, the liver is affected too. The stomach is affected also, where the impure blood is mixed with phlegm. Being involved in disease, the blood does not contribute to the regeneration of the seven bodily constituents. In turn the small intestine is affected, where the bile humor becomes involved. In the end the large intestine is affected along with the wind humor. This results in the full-blown dark-phlegm condition with the blood and all three humors affected.

The cold variety of dark-phlegm disorder is caused by the excessive intake of cold-natured, unfamiliar, or hard-to-digest foods. A lot of mucus is produced as a result. This weakens the fire-like wind and the digestive bile. The liver is then invaded by the undigested food material and becomes enlarged. In turn the blood is disturbed, and as with the heat variety of dark phlegm, the bodily constituents are no longer replenished. The accumulated undigested materials turn into phlegm and weaken the stomach. This variety is said to remain hidden in the body like a jackal.

General Diagnosis of Dark-Phlegm Disorders

The diagnosis of dark phlegm requires special care because of the involvement of multiple humors. The doctor may incorrectly diagnose poisoning, a hot or cold condition, or even a disease caused by the provocation of energy (elemental spirits). Early in the course of the disease, there appear signs and symptoms that indicate a disorder of the stomach and liver. Later on, various signs and symptoms appear as follows:

- The pulse is thick and full, but indistinct at the middle-finger positions. If cold is predominant, the pulse may be thready and slow.
- The urine is of mixed color or brownish, has some fume, a strong smell, and is dense and turbid; it may also be red-brownish or greenish.
- Symptoms that pertain to the stomach and liver, nausea but no vomiting, and dry, round, and purplish stools
- Cough producing purplish sputum with blood
- Sensation of heaviness and nausea with inability of the legs to support the body
- Fishy smell at the mouth and at the genitals
- Pain in the spinal joints, lower back, calves, nose, head, eyes, and bones, or pain and fluttering sensation at the back and flank
- Relief from massaging the spinal discs
- Tingling sensation all over the body
- Sensation of heat in the interior of the body
- After sweating, the patient might feel cold and have stomach cramps.

Contradictory symptoms may be present, such as aggravation after eating and also when hungry; aggravation both when exposed to cold and when exposed to heat; or the disease may appear suddenly and disappear suddenly. Symptoms generally are aggravated in the fall and in the spring.

Dark phlegm develops in three phases, which progress from the least to most serious:

- In the first phase, there is vomiting of hot and sour liquid.
- In the second phase, the disease matures and large amounts of yellow fluid can be seen when purgation or emesis (described below) is performed.
- In the final and most serious phase, there is vomiting of dark and sticky blood.

Changes related to diet and lifestyle may also be helpful when diagnosing dark-phlegm disorders. The illness is made worse with the intake of fresh cereal or pulses, stale food, old butter, noodle soup with meat, stale meat, sour foods, sour yogurt, greasy or heavy foods, and excessively hot or cold foods. Improvement can be seen on the intake of fresh meat, old cereal or pulses, mild yogurt, fish, light and smooth foods, and foods that are neither too warm nor too cold.

General Treatment of Dark–Phlegm Disorders

As for the treatment of each of the three humors, dark-phlegm conditions can be treated by dietary or lifestyle changes or using internal or external therapy.

Lifestyle and Diet

- For the hot variety of dark phlegm, the patient should eat fish, beef or pork, yogurt, buttermilk, and peas, and drink tea and cold water. Hot food and drinks should be avoided as well as strenuous physical activity.
- For the cold variety of dark phlegm, the patient should eat river fish, beef, mutton, and other warming food and drink, and avoid heavy, cooling, or hard-to-digest foods. Exposure to cold and sleeping during the daytime should be avoided. Hot fomentation therapy can be beneficial.

Aromatic Recipes

To alleviate dark phlegm, the main formula consists of equal parts of *a ru ra* (chebulic myrobalan) and *brag zhun* (mineral pitch). This treats all types of dark-phlegm conditions, especially where heat is present. Sugar and honey should be taken before, during, and after taking those medicines.

- In order to open up the channels of the lungs and liver, add *cu gang* (bamboo pith) and *gur gum* (safflower) to the main formula.
- To counteract and alleviate fever caused by dark phlegm, add the powder of *se 'bru* (pomegranate), *bse yab* (Chinese quince), *star bu* (sea buckthorn), *'u su* (coriander), *ma nu pa tra* (elecampane), *ut pal* (Himalayan poppy), and *pi pi ling* (long pepper).
- To treat blood and phlegm disorders, add *tig ta* (chiretta) and *ba sha ka* (Malabar nut tree).
- If there is heat in excess, one should add *gi waM* (elephant or ox gallstone) and *tsan dan dkar po* (white sandalwood).
- If there is cold in excess, add *dwa lis* (rhododendron) and *bca' sga* (fresh ginger).

Stone Recipes

The main recipe consists of *gangs thigs* (smithsonite), *a ru ra* (chebulic myrobalan), and *brag zhun* (mineral pitch) as the chief ("king") ingredients; *ba sha ka* (Malabar nut tree) and *re skon* (Nepalese fumewort) as the assisting ("queen") ingredients; *cong zhi* (calcite) as deputy ("prince") ingredient; and *ma nu pa tra* (elecampane), *'u su* (coriander), and *star bu* (sea buckthorn) as envoys ("cruel ministers"). As a vehicle, *ka ra* (white rock sugar), *bu ram* (raw cane sugar), and *sbrang rtsi* (honey) should be taken with the medicines.

- If the heart and the life channel are affected, add *dzA ti* (nutmeg), *a ga ru* (eaglewood), and *tsan dan dkar po* (white sandalwood) to the main recipe.

- If there is excess heat and the condition is of recent origin, add *gi waM* (elephant or ox gallstone), *tsan dan dkar po* (white sandalwood), *cu gang* (bamboo pith), *gur gum* (safflower), and *li shi* (clove) to the main recipe.
- If the lungs are affected, add *cu gang* (bamboo pith), *rgun 'brum* (raisin), *shing mngar* (licorice), and *dom mkhris* (bear bile) to the main recipe.
- If the dark-phlegm condition is caused by heat hidden in the hollow organs, add *bong nga dkar po* (white aconite), *dom mkhris* (bear bile), and *gser gyi me tog* (bolenggua) to the main recipe.
- If the joints and channels are poisoned by dark phlegm, add *rgyal po re ral* (fern), *phag khrag* (pig blood), and *skyer pa'i bar shun* (barberry root middle bark) to the main recipe.
- For upward-moving manifest dark phlegm, add *rgya skyegs* (shellac), *pu shel rtse* (noble dendrobium), and roasted rice to the main recipe.
- For downward-moving dark phlegm, add *da trig* (schisandra), *bya rkang* (larkspur), and *dug mo nyung* (kurchi) to the main recipe.
- For fixed dark phlegm, add *star bu* (sea buckthorn), *rgyam tshwa* (rock salt), and *sbrul gyi sha* (processed snake meat) to the main recipe.
- For hidden dark phlegm, add *dwa lis* (rhododendron), *se 'bru* (pomegranate), and other hot ingredients to the main recipe.

Herb Recipes

The following constitute the main treatment of dark phlegm by herb recipes: *pri yang ku* (nodding dragonhead), *khur mang* (dandelion), *se rgod bar shun* (middle bark of *Rosa sp.*), *star bu* (sea buckthorn), and *yung ba* (turmeric).

- If the dark-phlegm is at the confluence of heat and cold, *dwa lis* (rhododendron), *shing tsha* (cinnamon), *sug smel* (green cardamom), *ra mnye* (Solomon's seal), and *sle tres* (moonseed) should be added as a fine powder to the main formula and taken with *ka ra* (white rock sugar) as a vehicle and with hot or cold water.
- If the disease is marked by strong aggravation of the blood, *tsan dan dmar po* (red sandalwood), *cu gang* (bamboo pith), *gur gum* (safflower), *ma nu pa tra* (elecampane), and *'u su* (coriander) should be added to the main formula and taken with *ka ra* (white rock sugar).
- If there is flatulence and belching, the decoction of *rgyam tshwa* (rock salt), *bca' sga* (fresh ginger), *a ru ra* (chebulic myrobalan), and *pi pi ling* (long pepper) should be added to the main formula.

- If there is vomiting, add *gur gum* (safflower), *dom mkhris* (bear bile), *rgya skyegs* (shellac), *pu shel rtse* (noble dendrobium), *'bras yos* (parched rice), *ka ra* (white rock sugar), and *sbrang rtsi* (honey) to the main formula.
- If there is diarrhea, *cong zhi* (calcite), *re skon* (Nepalese fumewort), *da trig* (schisandra), *dug mo nyung* (kurchi), and another part of *pri yang ku* (nodding dragonhead) should be added to the main formula and taken with thin rice gruel.

Emesis

One of two emetic formulas may be used in the treatment of dark phlegm:

- *se 'bru* (pomegranate), *ma nu pa tra* (elecampane), *gur gum* (safflower), *pi pi ling* (long pepper), *sug smel* (green cardamom), *cong zhi* (calcite), and *ka ra* (white rock sugar)
- *se 'bru* (pomegranate), *star bu* (sea buckthorn), *skyu ru ra* (amla), *da trig* (schisandra), *skyer pa* (barberry), and *skyer 'bru* (barberry fruit)

The modifications below can be made to either formula above:

- If the vomitus is yellow, add *dug mo nyung* (kurchi) and give the powder of *tig ta* (chiretta), *shing mngar* (licorice), *'u su* (coriander), *ka ko la* (black cardamom), and *dom mkhris* (bear bile) mixed with *ka ra* (white rock sugar).
- An alternative modification for yellow vomitus is the decoction of *shing mngar* (licorice), *gser gyi me tog* (bolenggua), *tig ta* (chiretta), *se 'bru* (pomegranate), *btsod* (Indian madder), *'bri mog* (Tibetan groomwell), and *rgya skyegs* (shellac).
- If the vomitus is bright red, add *tsan dan dmar po* (red sandalwood), *gur gum* (safflower), *cu gang* (bamboo pith), *tig ta* (chiretta), *ut pal* (Himalayan poppy), *ba le ka* (birthwort), *skyu ru ra* (amla), *skyer pa'i bar shun* (barberry root middle bark), and *ka ra* (white rock sugar) to be taken with *rgya skyegs* (shellac) dissolved in warm water.
- If the vomitus is red, putrid, and smoky, add *se 'bru* (pomegranate), *btsod* (Indian madder), *'u su* (coriander), *sug smel* (green cardamom), *pi pi ling* (long pepper), *bse yab* (Chinese quince), *shing mngar* (licorice), and *dom mkhris* (bear bile) to be taken with *sbrang rtsi* (honey).

External Therapy

External therapies such as bloodletting, purgation, moxibustion, or fomentation can be selected based on the patient's condition and combined with any of the treatments described above.

Classification and Treatment by Location

Dark phlegm may be located in its natural place, i.e. the stomach, liver, or intestines; or it can affect the exterior of the body: muscles, skin, blood vessels, or joints; or the interior of the body: channels, blood, and internal organs.

Dark Phlegm in the Stomach

The signs and symptoms are similar to those of phlegm disorders: belching, vomiting, and discomfort after eating, indigestion, aggravation when alcohol is consumed, and aggravation in hot, humid, and cold weather.

- For the first phase of treatment, the decoction of *ma nu pa tra* (elecampane), *kaNDa ka ri* (two-flowered raspberry), *sle tres* (moonseed), and *sga skya* (galangal) should be given.
- Next the patient should be given the powder of *se 'bru* (pomegranate), *shing tsha* (cinnamon), *sug smel* (green cardamom), and *sga skya* (galangal). The following ingredients may also be added: *gur gum* (safflower), *ma nu pa tra* (elecampane), *'u su* (coriander), and *star bu* (sea buckthorn).

Dark Phlegm in the Liver

The signs and symptoms are similar to those of blood disorders, or the following: back pain, relief after massage, aggravation when exposed to heat, or aggravation after taking sour foods. The blood should be treated for this condition.

- First, the cold decoction of *tig ta* (chiretta), *ru rta* (costus), *ba sha ka* (Malabar nut tree), *ma nu pa tra* (elecampane), and *pu shel rtse* (noble dendrobium) should be given.
- Next, the powder of *gur gum* (safflower), *cu gang* (bamboo pith), *gi waM* (elephant or ox gallstone), *ut pal* (Himalayan poppy), *ba sha ka* (Malabar nut tree), *pri yang ku* (nodding dragonhead), and *brag zhun* (mineral pitch) should be given.
- Alternatively, the following powder may be given: *cu gang* (bamboo pith), *gur gum* (safflower), *li shi* (clove), *brag zhun* (mineral pitch), *tig ta* (chiretta), *pi pi ling* (long pepper), *a ru ra* (chebulic myrobalan), and *mtshal* (cinnabar).
- If there is no relief from the above therapies nor from bloodletting, then the patient should be given a pill of *dur byid* (spurge), *hong len* (picrorhiza grass), and *tsha la* (borax).

Dark Phlegm in the Small Intestine

The signs and symptoms are similar to those of bile disorders, e.g. yellow sclera and urine, as well as gurgling in the intestines. Bile is the predominant humor.

- The patient should be given the decoction of *tig ta* (chiretta), *ma nu pa tra* (elecampane), and *dug mo nyung* (kurchi).
- Alternatively, the decoction of *dug mo nyung* (kurchi), *bong nga dkar po* (white aconite), *li ga dur* (cranesbill), and *ba le ka* (birthwort) may be given.
- The patient should then be given the powder of *brag zhun* (mineral pitch), *dug mo nyung* (kurchi), *bong nga dkar po* (white aconite), *dom mkhris* (bear bile), *ma nu pa tra* (elecampane), *'u su* (coriander), *a ru ra* (chebulic myrobalan), *li ga dur* (cranesbill), and *ka ra* (white rock sugar).
- If there is no relief, purgation therapy should be given.

Dark Phlegm in the Large Intestine

The signs and symptoms are similar to those of wind affecting the intestines: gas with a strong smell, distention and gurgling in the intestines, abdominal swelling especially in the evening or after drinking sour liquids, alleviation when eating warming foods, and aggravation when eating cooling foods. The wind humor is predominant.

- The patient should be given the decoction of *ma nu pa tra* (elecampane), *kaNDa ka ri* (two-flowered raspberry), *sle tres* (moonseed), and *sga skya* (galangal).
- This powder should be given with warm water: *se 'bru* (pomegranate), *pi pi ling* (long pepper), *na le sham* (black pepper), *sman sga* (ginger), *dzA ti* (nutmeg), *sug smel* (green cardamom), *ka ko la* (black cardamom), *gur gum* (safflower), *shing tsha* (cinnamon), *zi ra dkar po* (cumin), *a ru ra* (chebulic myrobalan), *rgyam tshwa* (rock salt), *kha ru tshwa* (black salt), and *bu ram* (raw cane sugar).
- If there is pelvic pain and constipation, a mild enema may be given.

Dark Phlegm in the Exterior of the Body

Signs and symptoms are abnormal growth in the muscles, cold sensation in the skin, mud-like appearance of the skin, and swelling of the joints.

- If the skin is affected, there is a hot sensation in the skin.
- If the blood vessels are affected, they appear swollen, dark, and edematous, and there is a tingling sensation in the affected areas.

- If the joints are affected, movement is limited, and there is swelling and pain at the joints. Heavy, rich, and warming foods aggravate the symptoms.
- If the face is affected, there is stiffness and pain at the jaw, wasting of facial muscles, and relief of pain when the head is raised.

Dark Phlegm in the Interior of the Body

Dark phlegm invades the interior of the body through the liver, the channels, and the blood.

- If the channels are affected, there is stiffness of the joints.
- If it rises up to the head, there are symptoms at the head, including a sensation of heaviness, pain in the orbits, and nosebleed.
- If dark phlegm disturbs the heart, this will manifest as the heart being disturbed by the wind humor. There will be trembling, chest pain, insomnia, and aggravation after alcohol intake. Pain is not relieved when hot soup is eaten or when given moxibustion therapy.
- If dark phlegm affects the lungs, there is a sensation of heat and heaviness of the chest, and continuous cough with expectoration of purplish sputum with blood. Hot soup and bloodletting therapy provide no relief. Medicines generally useful for diseases of the lungs will not help either.
- If dark phlegm invades the spleen, there will be colicky pain in the upper-left abdominal quadrant, pain when exposed to heat, groaning, and a purple-colored face.
- If dark phlegm invades the kidneys, there is a sensation of heaviness at the feet and in the groin, furrows in the thighs, reddish urine, and the pulse is imperceptible at the kidney position.
- If the reproductive organs are affected by dark phlegm, there is a discharge of blood or pus from the genitals of the male or female patient.

Classification and Treatment on the Basis of Phase

The location of a phlegm condition progresses along with the severity of the illness. Thus the phlegm at first causes stickiness of the skin, grows in the muscles, produces stiffness of the channels, attaches itself to the bones, falls on the solid organs, gets submerged in the hollow organs, and finally "blossoms" in the sense organs (head, eyes, eyes, ears, nose, and tongue).

Hot Phase

When the disease is in the hot phase, the bile and the blood are especially affected. Signs and symptoms are a tight pulse, brownish urine with a strong smell and a lot of fume, a dry and rough tongue, a bitter taste in the mouth, poor appetite, a sensation of heaviness, sleepiness, greasy face, red and cloudy eyes, pain and spasm at the diaphragm, pain in the head, orbits, and forehead, and aggravation when exposed to heat or after eating sour or pungent foods.

- The decoction of *ru rta* (costus), *tig ta* (chiretta), *ba sha ka* (Malabar nut tree), *pu shel rtse* (noble dendrobium), and *ma nu pa tra* (elecampane) relieves acute symptoms of dark phlegm.
- The following powder may be given to the patient mixed with *ka ra* (white rock sugar): *tsan dan dkar po* (white sandalwood), *gi waM* (elephant or ox gallstone), *gur gum* (safflower), *cu gang* (bamboo pith), *ma nu pa tra* (elecampane), *'u su* (coriander), *ba sha ka* (Malabar nut tree), *ut pal* (Himalayan poppy), *re skon* (Nepalese fumewort), and *brag zhun* (mineral pitch).
- This powder may also be given mixed with *ka ra* (white rock sugar): *a ru ra* (chebulic myrobalan), *brag zhun* (mineral pitch), *re skon* (Nepalese fumewort), *kyi lce* (broad-leaf gentian), *bong nga dkar po* (white aconite), *spang rtsi do bo* (*Pterocephalus hookeri)*, and *pri yang ku* (nodding dragonhead).
- This powder may also be given mixed with *ka ra* (white rock sugar) and cold water: *tsan dan dkar po* (white sandalwood), *gi waM* (elephant or ox gallstone), *cu gang* (bamboo pith), *gur gum* (safflower), *li shi* (clove), *tig ta* (chiretta), *ba sha ka* (Malabar nut tree), *ru rta* (costus), *brag zhun* (mineral pitch), and *a ru ra* (chebulic myrobalan).
- Bloodletting is indicated.
- If the above treatments are not effective, purgation therapy should be given.

Hot–and–Cold Phase

The hot-and-cold phase occurs when the heat of blood and bile and the cold of wind and phlegm balance each other out. The digestive bile is blocked and invades the stomach and the intestines. The disease becomes that of a confluence of heat and cold. Because of its contradictory hot-and-cold nature, this condition is difficult or impossible to treat: cold treatment aggravates the cold aspect of the illness, and warming treatment aggravates the hot aspect. This condition, also called disturbed dark phlegm, may end with the patient's death.

Signs and symptoms: pain or spasm that can be constant or intermittent, with alleviation during the day and constant pain at night, pain when hungry, relief after fomentation therapy, dry skin, prominent veins, and disappointing results from intake of either cold or hot food and medicine.

- Cold substances are contraindicated. The patient may take *khre ma* (millet), which is both hot and cold. The following powder mixed with *ka ra* (white rock sugar) is very helpful: *se 'bru* (pomegranate), *ma nu pa tra* (elecampane), *star bu* (sea buckthorn), *pi pi ling* (long pepper), and *ba sha ka* (Malabar nut tree).
- Purgation should be effected using *dur byid* (spurge), *star bu* (sea buckthorn), *dung thal* (calcined conch shell), *sbrul gyi sha* (processed snake meat), *rgya tshwa* (ammonium chloride), and *bu ram* (raw cane sugar).
- If purgation gives no relief, then a mild enema should be given seven to nine times. This removes residual wind and empties the colon of blood.
- After a selection of the above treatments, moxibustion may be given.

Cold Phase

If phlegm and wind together are stronger than blood and bile together, the disease is marked by cold signs and symptoms: coldness and weakness of the entire body, poor digestion, belching, discomfort after eating, diarrhea, gas, intestinal rumbling, and discomfort after taking water or wine.

- Large amounts of the following decoction should be given: *rgyam tshwa* (rock salt), *bca' sga* (fresh ginger), *a ru ra* (chebulic myrobalan), and *pi pi ling* (long pepper).
- The following powder should be given mixed with *ka ra* (white rock sugar): *se 'bru* (pomegranate), *shing tsha* (cinnamon), *sug smel* (green cardamom), *sga skya* (galangal), *na le sham* (black pepper), *ma nu pa tra* (elecampane), *'u su* (coriander), and *sman sga* (ginger).
- Enema, moxibustion, and the intake of warm fluids are beneficial.
- Bloodletting, purgation, and being exposed to cold and wind are contraindicated.

Varieties of Dark Phlegm and Follow-up

The Oral Instruction Tantra gives a brief classification of nine varieties of dark-phlegm disorders loosely based on four pairs of opposing criteria:

- Dispersion, which may be (1) internal or (2) external (refer to the section describing treatment based on location)
- Aggravation *(rgyas)*, which entails (3) exudation (rdol, for which three subcategories are described) or (4) no exudation (ma rdol, the more common condition, for which general treatment principles apply)
- Excessive aggravation *('gyings)*, which may be (5) hidden *(gab*, for which three subcategories are described) or (6) manifest *(ma gab,* the more common condition, for which general treatment principles apply)
- Fixed dark phlegm *('dril)*, referring to (7) a recently acquired *(gsar pa)* or (8) a chronic *(rnying pa)* condition. A third category of fixed dark phlegm is known as (9) diffused dark phlegm *(zags pa)*.

The treatment of the varieties of dark phlegm is divided into the following sections:

- Obstructive and nonobstructive dark-phlegm conditions;
- Three subcategories of exudative, excessively aggravated dark phlegm *(rdol)*, namely upward moving, downward moving, and subdued (an alternative classification is described in the same chapter of the Oral Instruction Tantra as obstructive, nonobstructive, and subdued dark phlegm);
- The general treatment of hidden *(gab)*, excessively aggravated dark phlegm *('gyings)*; and
- Blood tumors, which can probably be classified as the end stage of fixed dark phlegm.

Follow-up treatment consists of the following:

- Very chronic dark phlegm
- Relapsing dark phlegm and prevention

The general formula for treatment on the basis of variety classification is as follows, subject to modifications: *gur gum* (safflower), *cu gang* (bamboo pith), *ut pal* (Himalayan poppy), *ba le ka* (birthwort), *tig ta* (chiretta), *skyu ru ra* (amla), and *skyer pa'i bar shun* (barberry root middle bark) as a powder mixed with *ka ra* (white rock sugar).

- Bloodletting on points that dispel wind is indicated.
- If the disease is very serious, one should resort to elimination therapies.
- If the head is affected, *dom mkhris* (bear bile), *tig ta* (chiretta), and *mtshe ldum* (ephedra) should be added to the main formula.

- If the heart is affected, *spos dkar* (frankincense), *dzA ti* (nutmeg), and *a ga ru* (eaglewood) should be added to the main formula.
- If the lungs are affected, *cu gang* (bamboo pith), *shing mngar* (licorice), and *mtshal* (cinnabar) should be added to the main formula.
- If the liver is affected, *brag zhun* (mineral pitch), *gur gum* (safflower), *ba sha ka* (Malabar nut tree), and *rgya skyegs* (shellac) should be added to the main formula.
- If the spleen is affected, *li shi* (clove), *gser gyi me tog* (bolenggua), and *pi pi ling* (long pepper) should be added to the main formula.
- If the kidneys are affected, *gla rtsi* (musk), *sug smel* (green cardamom), and *lcam pa* (mallow) should be added to the main formula.
- If the genitals are affected, *'bri mog* (Tibetan groomwell), *rgya skyegs* (shellac), and *btsod* (Indian madder) should be added to the main formula, or *zhu mkhan* (sapphireberry) could be substituted for *'bri mog* (Tibetan groomwell).

Afterward, bloodletting should be performed at the points appropriate for the organs affected. After the treatment has been completed, the patient should convalesce by bathing in natural springs.

Obstructive and Nonobstructive Dark Phlegm Conditions

If the blood vessels are obstructed, there is no bleeding. If there is no pain and the patient's body feels light, prognosis is favorable.

If the blood vessels are not obstructed, even after abundant emesis and purgation the secretion of red, black, or smoky fluids is uninterrupted. There will be no relief, and the patient will lose strength. If the patient loses appetite, the disease will be difficult to treat.

Upward–Moving Dark Phlegm

Aggravated *(rgyas)* upward-moving dark phlegm is treated as follows:

- It should be uprooted by giving the patient nourishing food.
- If that is not sufficient, massage and fumigation as well as bone soup, *bu ram* (raw cane sugar), and other foods that alleviate wind should be given.
- Taking care of protecting the seven bodily constituents, emetic therapy (as described in this chapter) should be given in order to remove the diseased blood and humors.
- If the seven bodily constituents are depleted and the blood is not obstructed, the patient should be given a light soup with rice, *skyu ru ra* (amla), *pu shel rtse* (khus khus grass), and *sbrang rtsi* (honey).

- The patient may be given a cold decoction of *tsan dan dkar po* (white sandalwood), *pu shel rtse* (khus khus grass), *ba le ka* (birthwort), *li da gur* (cranesbill), and *par pa ta* (fumitory).
- Calcined *pri yang ku* (nodding dragonhead) mixed with butter may also be helpful.
- Purgation may also be administered using *dur byid* (spurge), *a ru ra* (chebulic myrobalan), *ba ru ra* (beleric myrobalan), *skyu ru ra* (amla), *pri yang ku* (nodding dragonhead), and *pi pi ling* (long pepper) mixed with *sbrang rtsi* (honey).

To conclude the course of therapy, a thin gruel should be prepared with *se 'bru* (pomegranate), *skyu ru ra* (amla), and popped rice ground into a powder.

Downward-Moving Dark Phlegm

Aggravated *(rgyas)* downward-moving dark phlegm is treated in a manner similar to the upward-moving variety. The following additional modalities may also be helpful:

- If the seven bodily constituents are depleted, then *tha ram* (plantago), *bya rkang* (larkspur), and *rgya skyegs* (shellac) should be given.
- The following may be given to the patient: *da trig* (schisandra), *dom mkhris* (bear bile), *pri yang ku* (nodding dragonhead), and *re skon* (Nepalese fumewort) mixed with *ka ra* (white rock sugar).
- Alternatively, a rice gruel containing *re skon* (Nepalese fumewort), *cong zhi* (calcite), and *ka ra* (white rock sugar) may be given.
- The cold decoction of *ba sha ka* (Malabar nut tree), *pri yang ku* (nodding dragonhead), *tshur nag* (black alunite), *zhu mkhan* (sapphireberry), and concentrated extract of *skyer pa* (barberry) with *sbrang rtsi* (honey) may also be given.
- This formula may also be helpful: *a ru ra* (chebulic myrobalan), *ba ru ra* (beleric myrobalan), *skyu ru ra* (amla), *ka bed* (squash seed), *mon cha ra* (Himalayan oak acorn), and roasted rice flour mixed with *ka ra* (white rock sugar).
- Moxibustion is indicated.
- In order to replenish the blood, cow or goat milk boiled with *pu shel rtse* (khus khus grass) should be given as an enema.

Subdued Dark Phlegm

The signs and symptoms of aggravated *(rgyas)*, exudative, subdued dark phlegm are bleeding, red urine with bubbles, an empty fast pulse, discomfort in the area of the heart and lungs, heavy breathing, gooseflesh, a dull tongue, lips, and nails, a yellow face, distention on the side of the neck, trembling in the upper part of the feet, and thirst with a desire for cold drinks.

In general the blood is exhausted, and the patient may die. But if the illness subsides, the patient should be given goat milk boiled with sugar and butter at the time when wind is prevalent.

The patient should be given fresh meat, fresh butter, young wine or ale, *ka ra* (white rock sugar), *bu ram* (raw cane sugar), and *sbrang rtsi* (honey).

The patient should then take the white soup that expels wind (*dkar 'don*, described in the chapter on wind disorders) with the formula *cu gang bde byed chung* (Lesser Comforting Bamboo Pith): *cu gang* (bamboo pith), *gur gum* (safflower), *li shi* (clove), *se 'bru* (pomegranate), *ut pal* (Himalayan poppy), *pi pi ling* (long pepper), and *shing tsha* (cinnamon).

Hidden Dark Phlegm

Excessively aggravated (*'gyings*) hidden (*gab*) dark phlegm is characterized by excessive cold in the head and excessive heat in the hollow internal organs. Additional signs and symptoms are a fast, fine, and hidden pulse, greenish urine, a sensation of heaviness, nausea, loss of appetite, loss of the sense of taste, pain in the back and over the area of the liver, relief of symptoms after vomiting, aggravation of symptoms after fomentation therapy and after taking yogurt or buttermilk, relief of symptoms after intake of warm foods or other warming regimens, and indigestion with heartburn and dry stools.

This condition is divided into three subtypes: fixed and recent, fixed and chronic, and diffused.

- Signs and symptoms of fixed, recent, excessively aggravated (*'gyings*) hidden (*gab*) dark phlegm are strong and continuous colic pain, nausea, weakness, poor appetite, local sensations of heat, a fast, thready, and rapid pulse, reddish urine, and other serious acute symptoms.
- Signs and symptoms of diffused excessively aggravated (*'gyings*) hidden (*gab*) dark phlegm are facial swelling, pitting edema of the limbs, a variable pulse, and salivation accompanied by thirst. If the urine is hot, the prognosis is good. However, if there is a hidden tumor, the disease may reoccur after treatment has been completed.
- If, on the other hand, the condition is fixed and chronic, it is easy to treat.

The general approach to treating hidden dark phlegm is outlined as follows:

- The main formula is *dzA ti* (nutmeg), *sug smel* (green cardamom), *ka ko la* (black cardamom), *li shi* (clove), *cu gang* (bamboo pith), *gur gum* (safflower), and *cong zhi* (calcite) in a decoction.
- After the main treatment course, either purgation therapy or the slower-acting combination of *a ru ra* (chebulic myrobalan), *brag zhun* (mineral pitch), and *re skon* (Nepalese fumewort) should be given to the patient.
- Afterward, the main formula should be given again supplemented with *skyu ru ra* (amla), *ba sha ka* (Malabar nut tree), *ru rta* (costus), *bong nga dkar po* (white aconite), *bu ram* (raw cane sugar), and *sbrang rtsi* (honey) in warm water.
- If digestion is poor, *se 'bru* (pomegranate), *shing tsha* (cinnamon), *sug smel* (green cardamom), and *sga skya* (galangal) should be given. If there is a gurgling noise in the abdomen with diarrhea, then the patient should take less food when taking the medicine, and the medicine should be taken with warm water.
- If the disturbed humor "adheres like yogurt" (i.e. is very persistent), purgation therapy should be given. But if purgation is not feasible because of the patient's condition, the humor should be brought back to its normal location (stomach, liver, and intestines) and then eliminated.
- For purgation, a pill made of *dur byid* (spurge), *star bu* (sea buckthorn), *tsha la* (borax), and *bu ram* (raw cane sugar) should be given.
- To clear both heat and cold in excess, bone soup should be given with *rgyam tshwa* (rock salt) and *star bu* (sea buckthorn).

Dark Phlegm Resulting in a Tumor of the Blood

If the blood tumor is fixed, it should be reduced by giving calcined salt or a mixture of hot herbs with *cong zhi* (calcite). Fish, pork, and *sbrul gyi sha* (processed snake meat) are beneficial.

When the tumor ruptures, it becomes softer; the patient will lose appetite and the pulse and urine will show signs of heat. At that time, a pill should be made with *dur byid* (spurge), *rgyam tshwa* (rock salt), *star bu* (sea buckthorn), *sbrul gyi sha* (processed snake meat), and *bu ram* (raw cane sugar). This pill removes the waste products of the dissolving blood tumor.

Very Chronic Dark Phlegm

If the disease becomes very chronic, it is difficult to treat. Medication, bloodletting, and purgation should be employed. When the heat subsides and there is downward movement, the disease should be eliminated through purgation.

Relapsing Dark Phlegm and Prevention

Since dark phlegm is caused by a combination of humors, it is difficult to treat. Relapse is common, and treatment must be given over a long time. The analogy given is that of a gold container that is very dirty, and therefore must be scraped very gently so as not to wear it out; thus the seven bodily constituents must be protected. As soon as the illness begins to fade, nourishing foods should be given as support.

In order to prevent relapse, the following steps should be taken:

- Purgation should be resorted to by means of powder recipes.
- Moxibustion should be performed.
- The patient should refrain from harmful diets and behaviors, as indicated by the seasons, for a year or even more. In this way, the disease will not reoccur and the patient will be strong.

Fever Disorders

Fever disorders are described in general outline in Chapter 12 of the Oral Instruction Tantra and in more detail in subsequent chapters. This chapter represents a synthesis of chapters 12 to 22 of the original text. Chapters 23 to 27 of the Oral Instruction Tantra more clearly refer to hot disorders of infectious origin and are treated in the following chapter.

Contemporary translations render the term *tsha* as fever, but this entity is not identical to the condition described in Western medicine. While the authors prefer to translate *tsha* as the more abstract "heat," fever has been retained in most places for consistency with existing translations. Thus in this work the terms heat and fever are used interchangeably.

All disorders fall into the categories of hot and cold, but hot disorders are more common. Since hot disorders often resemble one another, they are easy to confuse and thus are somewhat complex to diagnose. Hot disorders can worsen very quickly and even lead to death.

General Diagnosis of Fever Disorders

The primary cause of hot disorders, based on the Buddhist view of illness, is an erroneous view of the self as actually existing, which leads to the arising of the five negative emotions of desire, hatred, indifference, pride, and jealousy. Of those, hatred increases the bile humor. If the bile humor's hot and sharp qualities increase beyond their normal level, the bile begins to attack the seven bodily constituents and the three excretions. This leads to a hot disorder.

Secondary causes of bile increase are:

- Season, climate, or inadequate treatment of an existing disease
- Provocations of energy either by elemental spirits or by *mamos*[9]
- A diet based on pungent, sour, salty, or very rich foods, including meat, molasses (treacle), alcohol, etc.
- Vigorous exercise, especially immediately after resting, or injury

General signs and symptoms of a hot disorder include:

- Tight, emergent, and rapid pulse
- Orange urine with a strong smell and a lot of fume

---

[9]. See the chapter on epidemic fever.

- Headache, fever
- A sour or bitter taste in the mouth
- Dry nostrils, an orange hue in the eyes
- Fixed, acute pain
- Yellow and salty-tasting sputum
- Strong thirst
- Diarrhea with blood and bilious fluids
- Panting
- Strong body odor
- Insomnia at night and sleepiness during the day
- Worsening of symptoms at noon, at midnight, and during digestion

In addition, exploratory treatment may aid in diagnosing a hot condition. If cooling foods and remedies or the corresponding lifestyle and climate changes improve the patient's condition, a hot disorder can be confirmed.

General Treatment of Fever Disorders

Treatment must be applied carefully, for there is always a risk of making the patient worse. Hot and cold conditions often present simultaneously. This means that heat and cold must be brought out and then treated separately. This is called separating heat from cold. No other approach is possible; if a fever is treated without first separating it from cold, the cold condition will remain for a long time, and so will the fever, although this may not create a life-threatening condition. Treating the cold first is easy, but proper timing must be observed in order not to endanger the patient. This is accomplished using *sle tres* (moonseed) for wind-related fever, *skyu ru ra* (amla) for blood-related fever, and *se 'bru* (pomegranate), *ma nu pa tra* (elecampane), and *sga skya* (galangal) together for phlegm-related fever. This approach is employed with turbid, unripe, or hidden fever.

A spread ailment must first be "gathered." The treatment must also be adjusted to the age of the patient and the state of the seven bodily constituents. The analogy is that one must not load a sheep with a load suitable for a horse. A child's bodily constituents have middling strength, while those of an adult are strongest. The elderly have the weakest constitution and are especially prone to wind. A child must be treated with care, as one would treat a relative. An adult must be treated forcefully, as one would treat an enemy. An older person should be treated "as one's own child," meaning, metaphorically, even more gently and carefully than when treating another person's child.

The strength of treatment depends on the chronicity of the condition. A recent fever must be treated quickly and forcefully like thunder, using purgation. This is the direct approach described in the next section. Chronic fever has the nature of a stain that has remained on a garment for a long time, and must be treated gradually and subtly, almost unnoticeably.

The following key principles summarize the approach to treating hot conditions:

1. Adjusting the treatment according to the age and strength of the patient
2. Selecting a treatment approach based on the chronicity of the illness
3. Selecting a treatment approach based on the humor affected:

   - For wind disorders, treatment must be nourishing as well as cooling.
   - For bile disorders, treatment must be fast and forceful.
   - For phlegm disorders, treatment is like removing ashes that cover burning embers.
   - For blood disorders, the fever must be gathered by administering a decoction in order to separate the diseased blood from the nutritive blood. Bloodletting must then be performed.
   - For lymph (*chu ser*)[10] disorders, treatment involves purgation and draining.

4. Treating the disorder based on the affected part of the body:

   - If the skin and flesh are affected, use cold water and steam baths.
   - If the channels and blood vessels are affected, the patient should be given a decoction to separate heat from cold, then bloodletting treatment.
   - If the solid organs are affected, herbs should be administered, followed by bloodletting.
   - If the bones are affected, treatment should consist of fomentation and medicinal baths.
   - If the hollow organs are affected, purgation is indicated.

5. Treating the strongest ailment first: if a humor is in excess but remains in its natural location, that humor should be treated first. Likewise if a humor goes out of its natural location, it should be treated in priority. If several humors are in excess, the strongest should be treated first.
6. Preparatory treatment in managing fever:

---

[10] The term *chu ser* represents a kind of residue of the blood. It has also been translated as "pus" or "serum."

- Unripe fever must be ripened.
- Hidden fever must be revealed.
- Very high fever must be treated without delay.
- Void fever must be treated by nourishing.
- Turbid fever is associated with an excess of lymph (chu ser) and must be dried before it is cooled.

7. The seventh principle deals with complex fever cases, i.e. disturbed fever, spread fever, epidemic fever, and fever that originates from poisoning. Toxic fever is said to be attached to the three humors. Its treatment must be subtle and applied to all three humors equally. Disturbed fever, spread fever, and epidemic fever are discussed elsewhere.

A mixed hot-and-cold disorder may be treated by whatever treatment improves the patient's condition. One must alternate cold and hot treatments between morning and evening.

Several pitfalls may affect the course of treatment. If the treatment of fever is too conservative (not strong enough), it will appear to work but will not root out the illness. The remaining fever will in time damage the seven bodily constituents. This may happen if the doctor is too confident about the outcome of treatment. Whatever one does when treating fever, one should be determined, patient, and not stop prematurely. In order to prevent side effects, the treatment should be rejuvenating as well. In order to correct the effects of the insufficient treatment of fever, one may prescribe cu gang (bamboo pith), gur gum (safflower), li shi (clove), and sug smel (green cardamom).

On the other hand, it is possible to give an excessively strong treatment, in which case wind and phlegm will attack the body like enemies, increase cold, and finally attack the life channel. In this case, moxibustion should be performed at the back points related to the heart channel and the life channel.

Other general recommendations include:

- Unripe fever should be increased so that it will follow its course.
- For fully developed fever, take more cold foods and drink.
- Toward the end of a course of treatment (when the body has been weakened by treatment or long illness), or if the patient is weak, fever may be associated with wind. Nourishing food should be given.
- If there is doubt about the nature of the disease, food that is likely to improve the condition should be given as exploratory treatment.

- If the treatment of fever was too forceful and cold developed as a result, one must increase the digestive heat.
- One should consider strengthening the seven bodily constituents if those appear weak.

If none of the above strategies is of any help, one may conclude that the illness is due to the patient's karma. The patient may benefit from performing meritorious deeds. A common practice among Tibetans is called animal release. People will purchase live animals from butcher shops or slaughterhouses, or otherwise rescue animals or fish from certain death, and release them where they can live out their normal life spans. This practice is said to lengthen the life of the practitioner or at least mitigate any karma leading to a shortened life span.[11]

Phases of Manifestation

Hot disorders, whether treated or untreated, may evolve from one phase to another. Each phase requires a different approach. For all but the simplest cases, therefore, the practitioner must be aware of the phase of a hot disorder before attempting treatment.

Unripe Fever

In this phase the fever does not manifest because wind and phlegm prevent it from "ripening" through their cold nature. Just as when green wood is put onto a fire, there is no blaze even though the wood continues to burn. The wind transports the fever through the seven bodily constituents while the phlegm suppresses the fever. If unripe fever is not treated skillfully, it can turn to hidden fever.

Predisposing factors are those of wind and phlegm, namely being of wind or phlegm constitution, being a child or an older patient, and related dietary and environmental conditions. Other causes include treating a fever prematurely, thus causing the fever to spread.

Signs and symptoms include a fast, thin, and mobile pulse, thick, turbid, and orange urine, white tongue with red dots, changing body temperature, yawning, stretching, lassitude, headache, a bitter taste in the mouth, headache, calf or arm pain, shivering, aversion to cold, agitated dreams, and worry.

Unripe fever is similar to hidden fever but with both the wind and phlegm humors affected. Giving the patient a cold medicine will make the disease worse.

[11.] For more details on this practice, see Foundation for the Preservation of the Mahayana Tradition 2005, cited in the bibliography.

In order to get rid of the wind and phlegm, a warming treatment must be given. The fever will not worsen but will become more amenable to treatment. The fever is made manifest by giving a decoction of *ma nu pa tra* (elecampane), *kaNDa ka ri* (two-flowered raspberry), *sle tres* (moonseed), and *sga skya* (galangal). This warming treatment is also appropriate for hidden fever. When the fever has been ripened, it may then be treated using cold remedies.

Hidden Fever

The main cause of hidden fever is cold and wind. This is often the result of treating an unripe fever using cold foods or medicine instead of helping it ripen. Treating hidden fever is similar to removing ashes from the top of burning embers.

Predisposing factors are living in a cold or damp area, being a child, and winter. The fever is mild and tends to stay in the lower part of the body, where wind usually resides. The stomach, heart, or kidneys may be affected.

Whether heat or cold predominates in the presentation gives rise to different treatment approaches. If cold is predominant, the pulse will be slower than expected, the urine will be pale with no change over time, and there will be a pale face, stiffness, poor appetite, runny nose, and mental dullness. There will also be amelioration when warm foods or drinks are taken.

If heat is predominant, there will be a fast and twisted pulse that feels like a rope spinning lengthwise under the skin, reddish urine that changes little or not at all, mental dullness, oily face, dry mouth after sleeping, a bitter taste in the mouth, poor appetite, occasional sweating, a sensation of heaviness in the head or in the whole body, red eyes, nosebleed, insomnia, sleepiness during the day, a feeling of oppression after being in the sun, fatigue when climbing stairs or slopes, and discomfort after taking cooling or warming foods.

The main difference between the two is the extent to which the ripening (first phase) of treatment must be applied. The practitioner must use clinical judgment to decide when to switch to the second phase of treatment.

The fever is made manifest by giving a decoction of *a ru ra* (chebulic myrobalan), *ba ru ra* (beleric myrobalan), *skyu ru ra* (amla), *ba le ka* (birthwort), *ut pal* (Himalayan poppy), *sle tres* (moonseed), *tig ta* (chiretta), *bong nga dkar po* (white aconite), *li ga dur* (cranesbill), and *ba sha ka* (Malabar nut tree). The ripening approach described in the treatment of unripe fever may also be used.

When the fever is manifest, it is reduced using the powder of *cu gang* (bamboo pith), *gur gum* (safflower), *li shi* (clove), *tig ta* (chiretta), *bong nga dkar po* (white aconite), *li ga dur* (cranesbill), and *ka ra* (white rock sugar). This formula may also be used at the end stage of treating unripe fever, i.e. when the fever is ripened.

Fully Developed Fever

Fully developed fever is attributed to the *mamos* and *dakinis*[12] being angry. It is not combined with wind or phlegm. As a result, the seven bodily constituents burn up like dry wood. Treatment is relatively straightforward and relies on a cooling diet and herbal medication. After the course of herbal treatment has been completed, bloodletting can be performed.[13]

Typical signs and symptoms include a fast pounding pulse, yellowish or reddish urine with a strong smell and a lot of fume, reddish or yellow abundant thick sputum, shortness of breath, sharp pains, dry mouth, discoloration of the teeth, a sensation of heaviness, poor appetite, thirst, a desire for cold foods, and sweating with a strong body odor.

Treatment proceeds in two phases. The first separates the diseased blood from the rest of the seven bodily constituents. The second phase destroys the heat. If the first phase of treatment is not performed, removing the heat may injure the seven bodily constituents.

- At first, the following decoction should be given: *tig ta* (chiretta), *sle tres* (moonseed), *skyu ru ra* (amla), and *ba sha ka* (Malabar nut tree). The liquid must be boiled down by two thirds and then allowed to cool down before drinking.
- Then the heat should be brought down with the decoction of *sle tres* (moonseed), *skyu ru ra* (amla), and *ba le ka* (birthwort). If the fever is very strong, one may add *hong len* (picrorhiza grass), *tig ta* (chiretta), and *ba sha ka* (Malabar nut tree).

Void Fever

In void fever the body is very weak, and the fever is not very strong. Cooling herbs and bloodletting are contraindicated. Void fever must be treated by nourishing. Later the fever may be removed by giving cooling herbs.

In order to diagnose void fever, which is associated with wind, the patient may be given bone soup seasoned with onion and garlic as exploratory treatment. This is called "detecting the fever."

It is desirable to pacify wind, which causes the bodily heat to leave its normal pathways and manifest as void fever. Old meat, old butter, barley ale, and *bu ram*

[12.] See the chapter on epidemic fever.

[13.] In practice, fully developed fever can amount to a life-threatening condition that warrants prompt biomedical referral.

(raw cane sugar) will all help alleviate void fever. This is called "redirecting the fever."

Chronic Fever

Chronic fever originates from a hot condition, such as dark phlegm or intoxication, that has lingered for many months or years. It may also be the result of an inappropriate diet or lifestyle. It is said that as a result of the heat being lodged in the body for a long time, it becomes so intermingled with the seven bodily constituents as to be inseparable from them. The analogies are rust on an iron vessel and an oil stain on cloth, both of which are hard to remove without causing damage. The condition may be present with or without wind.

General signs and symptoms are a thready pulse, reddish urine with a fume that persists a long time, oily face, sticky lips, dry mouth, difficulty swallowing, bloodshot eyes, tears, pale dry blotched skin, heart palpitations or trembling in the lungs upon movement, heat sensation over the shoulders, heaviness of the limbs, numbness of the extremities, desire for cold drinks, desire to stay in the shade especially at midday and at dusk, aggravation of symptoms after staying in a warm place, and light appetite.

In addition to the above, if wind is present there will be lack of strength, shivering, gooseflesh, spontaneous sweating, and joint pain.

If there is no wind present, treatment proceeds in six phases:

1. The treatment begins with separating the fever from the seven bodily constituents. Give the patient a cold decoction of *a ru ra* (chebulic myrobalan), *ba ru ra* (beleric myrobalan), *skyu ru ra* (amla), *tig ta* (chiretta), and *sle tres* (moonseed). This must be taken over a long time. When sweating and a sensation of lightness develop, it is time to move on to the next phase of treatment.

2. Then apply the plum-blossom needle as described in the chapter on bloodletting in part III of this book. This has the effect of weakening the fever.

3. Then the powder or pill of *tig ta* (chiretta), *hong len* (picrorhiza grass), *a ru ra* (chebulic myrobalan), *ba ru ra* (beleric myrobalan), *skyu ru ra* (amla), and *spang rtsi do bo (Pterocephalus hookeri)* should be given. This is said to uproot the fever.

4. The formula *ga bur 25* (Camphor 25) should be given with cold water along with either the decoction of *a ru ra* (chebulic myrobalan), *ba ru ra* (beleric myrobalan), and *skyu ru ra* (amla) or the decoction of *seng ldeng* (catechu tree). This furthers the treatment.

5. Next the fever is purged by giving the powder of *a ru ra* (chebulic myrobalan), *ba ru ra* (beleric myrobalan), *skyu ru ra* (amla), *lcum rtsa* (rhubarb), and *dur byid* (spurge) soaked in cow urine and mixed with honey for taste. This must be taken before meals. As this is bound to cause diarrhea sooner or later, the doctor should manage the patient accordingly.

6. In order to prevent relapse, the patient should be given the powder of *gi waM* (elephant or ox gallstone), *tsan dan dkar po* (white sandalwood), *cu gang* (bamboo pith), *li shi* (clove), *gur gum* (safflower), *ut pal* (Himalayan poppy), *sle tres* (moonseed), *brag zhun* (mineral pitch), and *ka ra* (white rock sugar).

If there is wind, medicinal butter made with *tig ta* (chiretta) should be given.

If both treatment approaches above fail, this suggests void fever, in which case the patient should be given a nourishing diet.

Turbid Fever

Turbid fever arises as a result of treating unripe fever incorrectly. It is considered a mixed fever and lymph *(chu ser)* disorder. Turbid fever may be caused by heat or cold. If cold is the cause of illness, the digestive system should be strengthened, then the fever can be treated. If heat is the main cause, a smooth purgative should be given.

Drying the heat is the approach taken to treat turbid fever. The foundation formula is a smooth purgative made of *a ru ra* (chebulic myrobalan), *ba ru ra* (beleric myrobalan), *skyu ru ra* (amla), *skyer pa* (barberry), *sle tres* (moonseed), *spos dkar* (frankincense), *thal ka rdo rje* (foetid cassia), *so ma rA dza* (aibika), and *seng ldeng* (catechu tree).

Disturbed Fever

Disturbed fever is mostly the result of inappropriate diet and lifestyle.

When treating disturbed fever, one must separate the fever from the healthy tissues to which it adheres, and then apply a purgative treatment.

Eliminating the heat in disturbed fever is accomplished using either of the two formulas below:

- *de wa (Corydalis melanochlora)*, *gser gyi me tog* (bolenggua), *par pa ta* (fumitory), *li ga dur* (cranesbill), and *a ru ra* (chebulic myrobalan)
- *hong len* (picrorhiza grass), *ba sha ka* (Malabar nut tree), *tsan dan dmar po* (red sandalwood), *spang rtsi do bo (Pterocephalus hookeri)*, and *skyu ru ra* (amla)

Spread Fever

Spread fever is thought to be caused by strenuous physical effort. It spreads through the seven bodily constituents, enters the blood, and emerges as a full-blown bile disorder. General symptoms of spread fever are pain in the strained part of the body, sprain, a thin, fast, and twisted pulse, reddish strong-smelling urine, a bright oily face, difficult movement, and being startled easily.

Spread fever may be internal or external. Internal spread fever may affect the heart, lungs,[14] liver, diaphragm, spleen, kidneys, stomach, large intestine, small intestine, gallbladder, bladder, or seminal vesicle. External spread fever may affect the bones, blood vessels and channels.

Mixed hot and cold disorders where cold is dominant, left untreated, may spread to the whole body and become turbid. The wind is like a commander that dispatches the disease throughout the channels; all spread disease is caused by wind. The disease must be gathered prior to the main treatment; otherwise the treatment will not be tolerated.

When treating spread fever, one must be careful with the seven bodily constituents. Treatment must be performed in three stages. First, the wind must be stopped so that the disease does not spread further. Next, the disease must be gathered. Finally, the treatment itself can be given, by which time it is as simple as putting out fire with water. If gathering the disease is difficult, purgation and medicinal baths should be used. If that is not successful, whichever organ is affected should be treated.

The general treatment approach is to gather the heat by using either of the two formulas below. Suitable modifications should be made depending on where the fever has spread.

- *ma nu pa tra* (elecampane), *kaNDa ka ri* (two-flowered raspberry), *sle tres* (moonseed), *sga skya* (galangal), *a ru ra* (chebulic myrobalan), *ba ru ra* (beleric myrobalan), and *skyu ru ra* (amla)
- *kaNDa ka ri* (two-flowered raspberry), *btsod* (Indian madder), *ba sha ka* (Malabar nut tree), and *bu ram* (raw cane sugar)

Fever of Infectious Origin

When treating epidemic fever, one must take it away and release it like a bird. Epidemic fever is described in the next chapter.

[14.] Further research is needed to confirm whether spread fever in the lungs corresponds to the modern biomedical diagnosis of tuberculosis.

Treatment Regimens for Heat Conditions

The internal treatment of hot conditions is either purgative or nonpurgative, as described below. The practitioners of old were very hesitant to administer external therapies, because those affect the various winds that circulate in the body and thus could disturb meditation. External therapies are therefore given as a last resort. Six external therapies may be given in the treatment of hot conditions:

- Bloodletting removes impure blood from the blood vessels.
- Steam bath removes heat through the pores of the skin.
- Fomentation relieves pain quickly but not over the long term.
- Medicinal baths are used to treat turbid fever.
- Cold-water therapy treats external heat conditions.
- Moxibustion reveals hidden fever.

Nonpurgative Treatments

If there is doubt whether the disease is of cold or hot nature, one may give the decoction of *go snyod* (caraway), *sman sga* (ginger), and *dzA ti* (nutmeg).

For turbid fever, this decoction may be given: *a ru ra* (chebulic myrobalan), *ba ru ra* (beleric myrobalan), *skyu ru ra* (amla), *skyer pa* (barberry), *sle tres* (moonseed), *spos dkar* (frankincense), *thal ka rdo rje* (foetid cassia), *so ma rA dza* (aibika), and *seng ldeng* (catechu tree).

This foundation formula may be given as a powder with modifications as required: *g.ya' kyi ma* (golden saxifrage), *re skon* (Nepalese fumewort), *sro lo dkar po (Pegaeophyton scapiflorum)*, *pri yang ku* (nodding dragonhead), *par pa ta* (fumitory), *sum cu tig* (Lhasa saxifrage), *yu gu shing nag po* (elderberry), *gang gA chung (Gentiana urnula)*, *dar ya kan*,[15] *tsher sngon* (blue poppy), *myang rtsi spras* (goldthread), *spang rgyan* (small-leaf gentian), *sgong thog pa* (wallflower), *khur mang rtsa ba* (dandelion root), *'om bu* (German tamarisk), *stab seng* (Korean ash), *byi tsher* (cocklebur), and *bya rgod spos* (larkspur).

- For epidemic fever, double the dosage of *par pa ta* (fumitory).
- For disturbed fever, add two parts of *spang rtsi do bo (Pterocephalus hookeri)*.
- For blood-related fever, add two parts of *hong len* (picrorhiza grass).
- For bile-related fever, add two parts of *tig ta* (chiretta).

The above formula is like water poured onto a pyre.

[15.] The term *dar ya kan* may refer to one of twenty-five possible cooling herbs (Pasang Yonten Arya 1998), or it may refer more specifically to *khrag khrog pa (Lepidium apetalum)*.

For strong fever, the following powder of aromatic herbs should be made: *ga bur* (camphor), *tsan dan dkar po* (white sandalwood), *cu gang* (bamboo pith), *tsan dan dmar po* (red sandalwood), *gi waM* (elephant or ox gallstone), *hong len* (picrorhiza grass), *tig ta* (chiretta), *ba sha ka* (Malabar nut tree), and *bong nga dkar po* (white aconite).

For moderate fever, this powder is effective: *tsan dan dkar po* (white sandalwood), *tsan dan dmar po* (red sandalwood), *gur gum* (safflower), *ut pal* (Himalayan poppy), *hong len* (picrorhiza grass), *li ga dur* (cranesbill), *gi waM* (elephant or ox gallstone), *tig ta* (chiretta), and *ba sha ka* (Malabar nut tree).

For mild fever, give the powder of *gi waM* (elephant or ox gallstone), *cu gang* (bamboo pith), *gur gum* (safflower), *ut pal* (Himalayan poppy), *ba sha ka* (Malabar nut tree), *ba le ka* (birthwort), *hong len* (picrorhiza grass), *tig ta* (chiretta), *li ga dur* (cranesbill), and *bong nga dkar po* (white aconite).

For fever associated with wind, this powder is effective: *a ga ru* (eaglewood), *cu gang* (bamboo pith), *gur gum* (safflower), *li shi* (clove), *dzA ti* (nutmeg), *sug smel* (green cardamom), *ka ko la* (black cardamom), *ru rta* (costus), *sle tres* (moonseed), *sgog thal* (calcined garlic), and *ka ra* (white rock sugar).

For fever with phlegm, this powder may be used: *cu gang* (bamboo pith), *gur gum* (safflower), *li shi* (clove), *ut pal* (Himalayan poppy), *se 'bru* (pomegranate), *pi pi ling* (long pepper), and *shing tsha* (cinnamon).

- For chronic fever affecting the lungs, add *rgun 'brum* (raisin) and *shing mngar* (licorice).
- For hidden chronic fever, add *rgun 'brum* (raisin), *shing mngar* (licorice), *tsan dan dkar po* (white sandalwood), and *gi waM* (elephant or ox gallstone).

For strong chronic fever, the patient may benefit from the formula *ga bur 25* (Camphor 25).

For moderate chronic fever, prepare the powder of *tsan dan dkar po* (white sandalwood), *cu gang* (bamboo pith), *gur gum* (safflower), *li shi* (clove), *dzA ti* (nutmeg), *sug smel* (green cardamom), *ka ko la* (black cardamom), *ba le ka* (birthwort), *rgya tig* (chiretta), *hong len* (picrorhiza grass), *ga bur* (camphor), *ut pal* (Himalayan poppy), *'bu su hang* (alfalfa), *gi waM* (elephant or ox gallstone), the "three *ge sar*" (one part each of the three different parts of the silk cotton tree flower), *shing mngar* (licorice), and *ru rta 'bras* (costus seed).

For mild chronic fever, use this variation: *gi waM* (elephant or ox gallstone), *cu gang* (bamboo pith), *gur gum* (safflower), *li shi* (clove), *dzA ti* (nutmeg), *sug smel* (green cardamom), *ka ko la* (black cardamom), *ba le ka* (birthwort), *rgya tig* (Indian chiretta), *hong len* (picrorhiza grass), *ga bur* (camphor), *ut pal* (Himalayan poppy), *'bu su hang* (alfalfa), a higher dosage of the "three *ge sar*" (one part each of the three different parts of the silk cotton tree flower), *shing mngar* (licorice), *ru rta 'bras* (costus seed), and *brag zhun* (mineral pitch).

When the three humors are involved, use the following powder: *gur gum* (safflower), *tsan dan dkar po* (white sandalwood), *cu gang* (bamboo pith), *hong len* (picrorhiza grass), *ba sha ka* (Malabar nut tree), *bong nga dkar po* (white aconite), *tig ta* (chiretta), and *gi waM* (elephant or ox gallstone).

- For disturbed fever, add *tsan dan dmar po* (red sandalwood), *shing mngar* (licorice), *ru rta* (costus), and *skyu ru ra* (amla).
- For epidemic fever, add *gser gyi me tog* (bolenggua), *skra bzang zil pa (Corydalis impatiens), li ga dur* (cranesbill), *de wa (Corydalis melanochlora), spang rtsi do bo (Pterocephalus hookeri),* and *bong nga dkar po* (white aconite).
- If the heart is affected, add *dzA ti* (nutmeg) and *a ga ru* (eaglewood).
- If the lungs are affected, add *a krong* (sandwort) and *shing mngar* (licorice).
- If the liver is affected, add *ut pal* (Himalayan poppy) and *brag zhun* (mineral pitch).
- If the spleen is affected, add *pi pi ling* (long pepper).
- If the kidneys are affected, add *sug smel* (green cardamom).
- If the stomach is affected, add *bong nga dkar po* (white aconite).
- If the bile is affected, add *gser gyi me tog* (bolenggua).
- If the lymph *(chu ser)* is affected, add *gla rtsi* (musk).
- If there is inflammation, add *gla rtsi* (musk) and *gu gul* (myrrh).

Purgation

Purgation requires three stages. The first stage aims at transforming the fever condition into one most amenable to treatment by purgation:

- Unripe fever should be ripened.
- Scattered fever should be gathered.
- In wind-related fever, the wind should be pacified.
- Hidden fever should be revealed.
- If the digestive heat is insufficient, it should be augmented.
- If the fever is very strong, it should be subdued first.

The above preliminaries employ techniques previously discussed.

The main purgative formula is a powder made of the following herbs: *thar nu* (Wallich spurge), *khron bu (Euphorbia stracheyi), hong len* (picrorhiza grass), *lcum rtsa* (rhubarb), *gser gyi me tog* (bolenggua), *khur mang* (dandelion), and *ka ra* (white rock sugar).

- If one is certain that the fever is ripe, one may add *ga bur* (camphor) and *gi waM* (elephant or ox gallstone).
- If the hollow organs are affected, add *brag zhun* (mineral pitch) and *dug mo nyung* (kurchi).
- If a previous purgation therapy was unsuccessful, add *tsha la* (borax) and *gur gum* (safflower).

If, as a result of the therapy, the stools come out reddish yellow and the patient's overall condition improves, the therapy was successful. Purgation may then be discontinued.

Prior to applying the concluding stage of treatment, the stools must come out as described above. If they do not, treatment must be continued; otherwise the condition will spread like wildfire. In the last stage of treatment, the patient must be given a little *tsam pa* (roasted barley flour) in cold water, rice noodles, or whey to be taken before meals. This has a cooling action, helps suppress the wind, and supports the digestive system. Afterward, warm foods may be given.

Bloodletting

There exist seven contraindications to bloodletting therapy:

- Unripe fever, which risks turning into turbid fever upon bloodletting
- Contagious fever, which may spread to the internal organs
- Disturbed fever: the pure blood must be separated from the impure blood prior to bloodletting. If not, the seven bodily constituents will be depleted, and wind will increase. This will scatter the fever, the impure blood will remain, and the fever will also remain.
- Void fever: if bloodletting is applied, wind and pain will increase. The patient should instead be given cool, nourishing foods. After that, bloodletting may be attempted.
- Inflammatory fever (fever associated with inflammation of tissues or wounds): if the fever is treated this way, the remaining blood will invade the life channel and cause the patient to die.
- Toxic fever: this is the result of the patient taking too much medicine, which has become toxic. If toxic fever is treated by bloodletting, the fever will remain. Instead, the patient should be treated by decoction and then given plum-blossom needle treatment. This technique is described in the chapter on bloodletting.
- If the patient's seven bodily constituents are weakened, bloodletting will weaken the patient even more. This would lead to a situation similar to the contraindication of disturbed fever, only much more serious.

When the fever has been fully ripened and fully separated is when the patient can benefit most from bloodletting. Failure to perform bloodletting in that case would be tantamount to negligence because of the loss of a valuable healing opportunity. If there is hidden fever, it should be revealed prior to bloodletting. If the fever is chronic, bloodletting should be very light and slow.

Steam Baths

Steam baths are an effective way to bring fever down. The steam may be of water or of a decoction of the appropriate cooling herbs. Steam bathing can be beneficial in the following cases:

- Unripe fever, if it is not too strong
- Void fever, if the therapy is supplemented by nourishing methods, e.g. bone soup
- Chronic fever
- Contagious fever, to separate the fever from the skin, bones, or flesh

Contraindications for steam bathing are:

- Strong unripe fever: sweat will not come out, but instead the fever will be disturbed and scattered throughout the body.
- If the patient's seven bodily constituents are weak, steam bathing will increase the wind and further deplete the seven bodily constituents.

Therapy is effective if the sweat induced by the steam bath has a strong smell.

Fomentation

Fomentation is described at the end of the section on therapeutics.

Medicinal Baths

Medicinal baths can be either natural or artificial. An artificial medicinal bath is made by pouring a decoction of the appropriate herbs into a bathtub. Natural baths refer to natural springs whose waters are considered therapeutic. Hot springs are very common in Tibet. Different types of hot springs are:

- Hot springs in areas rich in *cong zhi* (calcite) benefit acute phlegm, dark phlegm, arthritis, and bone disorders.
- Hot springs in areas rich in *brag zhun* (mineral pitch) benefit acute stomach, liver, and kidney problems and urinary trouble.

- Hot springs in areas rich in *mu zi* (sulfur) treat skin problems, lymph *(chu ser)* disorders, and illnesses caused by elemental provocations.
- Hot springs in areas rich in *ldong ros* (realgar) benefit lymph *(chu ser)* and skin disorders.
- Hot springs in areas rich in a mixture of minerals tend to exhibit properties associated with the preponderant mineral.

All the above are ineffective for fever affecting the skin, channels, flesh, and bones and for scattered fever.

Cold–Water Therapy

The best form of cold-water therapy is to enter a waterfall. The main indication is heat on the surface of the body. Such exposure will prevent the heat from getting worse. If the fever is scattered, it will be gathered. High fever will be reduced the way water is poured onto fire. High chronic fever and fever associated with wind will likewise be reduced. Cold-water therapy is contraindicated for unripe fever.

Moxibustion

Moxibustion or fire therapy prevents heat from being scattered. In relation to the treatment of fever, six kinds of condition benefit from fire therapy:

- Bile-related fever scattered in the blood vessels
- Wind that may arise at the concluding stage of the treatment of fever
- Contagious fever accompanied with wind of the shivering or panting type
- Inflammation of the flesh
- Cold that may arise at the end of the treatment of fever
- To prevent the increase of void fever

At the Threshold between Heat and Cold

When the treatment of a hot disorder nears its conclusion, it is possible that the condition reverts from a hot disorder to a cold one. This point is called the juncture between the mountain and the plain. If this stage is not recognized, further treatment can harm the patient.

Preventing the Arising of a Wind Disorder

Toward the end of the treatment of a fever condition, certain factors predispose the arising of a wind disorder:

- A wind constitution, or an elderly patient

- A hot disorder that affects areas where the wind resides (hips, joints, skin, ears, or large intestine)
- Additional mental factors that may disturb the wind humor
- Overzealous treatment using cold medicines, bloodletting, or purgation

When wind first arises, this may give rise to signs and symptoms that resemble those of a hot disorder, such as a fast pulse, reddish urine, fever, thirst, dry mouth, etc. At this stage it would be dangerous to continue treating the patient with cold medicine. Instead, a supportive diet should be given to prevent the arising of the wind humor. Finding the exact time to begin this diet is delicate because if it is given too early, it may increase the heat condition. The practitioner must be on the lookout for signs of wind amidst signs of improvement of the hot condition. Telling signs include large bubbles in the urine, an empty pulse, a dry and rough tongue, etc.

Preventing the Arising of a Cold–Bile Disorder

Toward the end of the treatment of a fever condition, certain factors predispose the arising of a cold-bile disorder:

- A bile constitution, or an adult patient
- A hot disorder that affects areas where the bile resides (liver, blood, sweat, eyes, or small intestine)
- Excessive intake of meat or alcohol, oversleeping, and strenuous physical activity

Such a cold-bile disorder could be confused as residual fever, but further cold treatment would aggravate the condition rather than improve it. Symptoms include increased body temperature, dry mouth, mental fogginess, spontaneous sweating, a good appetite, little thirst, disturbed sleep, irregular breathing, a tight superficial pulse combined with a loose deep pulse, orange urine, and a tongue reddish at the edge with a yellow coat. While this condition may be brought about by dietary excess, restricting the diet could conversely bring about a wind disorder as explained above.

Preventing the Arising of a Phlegm Disorder

Toward the end of the treatment of a fever condition, certain factors predispose the arising of a phlegm disorder:

- A phlegm constitution where cold is predominant, or a child patient

- A hot disorder that affects areas where the phlegm resides (throat, chest, lungs, head, nutritive essence, flesh, fat, stomach, or kidneys)
- Excessive cold treatment causing the fever to spread throughout the body

Symptoms of a phlegm disorder arising include a slow pulse, bluish urine, frequent urination, poor appetite, wet tongue, little thirst, swelling, pale face, and poor digestion. If a cold diet had been prescribed to address the hot disorder, discontinuing the diet would cause the hot disorder to arise again. Instead of just stopping the cold diet, the diet should be made warm and nutritious.

EPIDEMIC FEVER

This chapter concerns the treatment of contagious or epidemic fever in general, as described in Chapter 23 of the Oral Instruction Tantra. The Oral Instruction Tantra also contains chapters on specific infectious diseases:

- Smallpox (Chapter 24);
- Enteric or typhoid fever (Chapter 25);
- Diphtheria (Chapter 26);
- Catarrh or influenza (Chapter 27);
- Diseases caused by parasites (Chapter 50); etc.

These chapters are beyond the scope of this work and are therefore not described in detail.

According to the tradition, contagious fever is caused by a microorganism called *par pa ta,* whose nature is that of bile. It is described as having the head of a lizard, a big mouth, a long tail, and many legs like a centipede, which account for its velocity: it can traverse the entire body in a single instant. Another explanation for epidemic fever is the anger of the *mamos,* fierce female deities that causes illness when irritated, and *dakinis,* female Buddhist deities. Chapter 23 of the Oral Instruction Tantra quotes this ancient Buddhist prophecy:

> At the end of the last five hundred years [when the dharma degenerates],
> Because of their desirous nature, people will take to doing whatever they
>   like.
> *Vajra* brothers and sisters will quarrel among themselves,
> Monastics will fight each other,
> Bons, Buddhists, and others will curse one another,
> Lay followers of the doctrine will go against their principles and destroy
>   one another.
> At that time, the *mamos* and *dakinis* will be upset
> And send clouds of diseases previously unknown,
> Such as epidemics, enteric fever, throat inflammation, anthrax, and
>   plagues.

A modern Buddhist explanation is that lack of contentment leads people to an excess of worldly pursuits and to behavior inconsistent with that recommended for the season. Other causative factors are strenuous exercise, living in an area where there are strong smells, anger, fear of the environment (for example being preoccupied with food contaminants), and an irregular diet. This results in disruption and pollution of the environment. That pollution serves as a breeding ground for the pathogens through which illness takes place.

General Treatment of Epidemic Fever

Epidemic fever can be differentiated according to the stage of illness: early, middle, or late.

Early–Stage Epidemic Fever

At this stage, the fever is not considered fully developed. Signs and symptoms are cold shivers, headache, pain at the feet and at the joints, sensation of heaviness, inertia, disturbed dreams, yawning, hearing loss, delirium, desire to stay warm, aggravation of the symptoms in the early hours of the night, bitter taste in the mouth, rapid and mobile pulse, and turbid urine.

- The patient's diet and lifestyle should be neutral, i.e. producing neither heat nor cold.
- The following decoction may be given: *ma nu pa tra* (elecampane), *kaNDa ka ri* (two-flowered raspberry), *sle tres* (moonseed), and *sga skya* (galangal).
- This decoction may also be given: *sle tres* (moonseed), *kaNDa ka ri* (two-flowered raspberry), *a ru ra* (chebulic myrobalan), *ba ru ra* (beleric myrobalan), and *skyu ru ra* (amla).

Middle–Stage Epidemic Fever

If the fever is ripe, signs and symptoms are a sensation of heaviness, strong-smelling perspiration, yellow sclera, dark tongue or lips, headache, thirst, a downcast mental state, reddish urine with a strong smell and a lot of sediment, and a thin, tight, and rapid pulse.

- The treatment for middle-stage epidemic fever is sudorific therapy, which is accomplished by giving the decoction of *tig ta* (chiretta), *gser gyi me tog* (bolenggua), *de wa (Corydalis melanochlora), par pa ta* (fumitory), *li ga dur* (cranesbill), and *a ru ra* (chebulic myrobalan).
- If there is high fever, add to the above *ga bur* (camphor), *gi waM* (elephant or ox gallstone), *cu gang* (bamboo pith), *gur gum* (safflower), *bong nga dkar po* (white aconite), and *ka ra* (white rock sugar), and increase the dosage of *tig ta* (chiretta).

- If there is mild fever with yellowish sclera and urine, the treatment is purgation by means of the following mixture: *a ru ra* (chebulic myrobalan), *ba ru ra* (beleric myrobalan), *skyu ru ra* (amla), *dur byid* (spurge), *pi pi ling* (long pepper), *nA ga ge sar* (silk cotton tree), *sbrang rtsi* (honey), and *ka ra* (white rock sugar). This formula is effective for recent and long-standing epidemic fevers. For the same condition, sprinkling therapy and a cooling lifestyle and diet are recommended.
- In fully developed fever, yogurt should be avoided (this applies to most epidemic-fever disorders). If the fever has lasted more than thirteen days, this formula is like *amrita*[16] to the patient. Refer to the section in the previous chapter ("Fever Disorders") that pertains to fully developed fevers.

Late–Stage Epidemic Fever

The late stage of epidemic fever typically is a condition bordering between heat and cold. The practitioner should clearly distinguish the late stage from the early stage of contagious fever, which can look similar. The signs and symptoms of late-stage epidemic fever are similar to those of void fever: pain, especially at the hips, in the lumbar area, and in the bones in general; abundant sweating; insomnia; confusion; buzzing in the ears; dry and reddish tongue; retching; slurred speech; trembling; and hot sensations on the skin.

Exploratory treatment should be given to determine the humor involved. Improvement after taking bone soup indicates a wind condition. Improvement after taking a decoction of *tig ta* (chiretta) indicates a bile condition. Improvement after taking *rgyam tshwa* (rock salt) in hot water indicates a phlegm condition. Because of the similarity of late-stage epidemic fever with borderline hot-and-cold disorders, the treatment principles explained for the latter also apply to the former.

The principal treatment consists of the following herbs, with modifications based on the patient's condition: *sgog thal* (calcined garlic), *srad dkar* (locoweed), *snya lo (Polygonum sp.),* and *kyi lce* (broad-leaf gentian). If the condition is severe, all the ingredients should be calcined (separately) in a covered pan.

- If there is headache, add calcined *a ru ra* (chebulic myrobalan).
- For nosebleed, add calcined *mtshe ldum* (ephedra).
- For cough, add calcined *rgya skyegs* (shellac).
- If there is rib pain, add calcined *ma nu pa tra* (elecampane).
- If the sclera and urine are yellowish, add calcined *ri sho* (leopard plant).

---

[16] An elixir of longevity.

- For fever affecting the joints, add calcined *rta lpags (Lamiophlomis rotata)*.
- For constipation, add calcined *ra sug* (campion).
- For frequent urination, add calcined *gze ma* (puncture vine).
- If the contagious fever is associated with wind, take the main formula above with bone soup.

Treatment Based on Location

The following section describes the disease as it progresses from the surface to the interior of the body. Each aspect has a recommended treatment as a well as contra-indications. In general, failure to apply the correct treatment results in the disease being driven deeper inside or becoming harder to treat.

Pores of the Skin Affected by Epidemic Fever

Signs and symptoms: weakness, poor appetite, skin painful to the touch, goose-flesh, or sensation of hair standing on end

- Treatment of this condition should begin by fasting and drinking hot water. Cold food and medicine should be avoided because this will make it difficult for the fever to ripen. The diet and lifestyle should not be nourishing (the kind used in the treatment of wind) because this will make the fever attach itself to the bones.
- If, after fasting, the fever has ripened while remaining in the skin, this decoction can be given: *ma nu pa tra* (elecampane), *kaNDa ka ri* (two-flowered raspberry), *sle tres* (moonseed), and *sga skya* (galangal).
- If the fever has become strong, this decoction should be used instead: *a ru ra* (chebulic myrobalan), *ba ru ra* (beleric myrobalan), *skyu ru ra* (amla), and *sle tres* (moonseed).
- Moxibustion is contraindicated because it will drive the fever into the interior of the body. Bloodletting and purgatives are also contraindicated. If the fever was disturbed as a result of incorrect treatment, it will develop the qualities of a wind illness. However, sudorific therapy is contraindicated because it will drive the fever into the channels.

Channels and Blood Vessels Affected by Epidemic Fever

Signs and symptoms: sudden, transient sharp pains, downcast mental state, thirst, bitter taste in the mouth, reddish and turbid urine

The treatment consists of a powder of *cu gang* (bamboo pith), *gur gum* (safflower), *li shi* (clove), *dzA ti* (nutmeg), *sug smel* (green cardamom), *ka ko la* (black cardamom), *ba sha ka* (Malabar nut tree), *li ga dur* (cranesbill), and *ka ra* (white rock sugar) to be taken with food and drink of a cooling nature. Cooling herbs such as *ma nu pa tra* (elecampane), *sle tres* (moonseed), etc. should be avoided because they may reduce the patient's appetite. Moreover, eating rich, oily foods or performing moxibustion will disturb the fever and drive it deeper into the blood and channels, thereby making the disease harder to treat.

Muscles Affected by Epidemic Fever

Signs and symptoms: disorientation, sensation of heaviness, fever, desire to stay in the cold, apathy

This powder should be given to the patient: *gi waM* (elephant or ox gallstone), *cu gang* (bamboo pith), *gur gum* (safflower), *li shi* (clove), *a ru ra* (chebulic myrobalan), and *ka ra* (white rock sugar). This formula is cooling and smooth. Sudorific therapy is recommended.

Moxibustion is contraindicated because it will increase pain. Bloodletting is contraindicated because puncturing the blood vessels will cause bleeding for a long time (as opposed to the normal situation where bleeding stops spontaneously after the appropriate amount of blood has been drawn). Giving the patient a decoction is contraindicated, especially if it contains *ga bur* (camphor), because that will drive the fever into the channels and disturb the wind. The wind would then disturb the entire body.

Hollow Organs Affected by Epidemic Fever

Signs and symptoms: poor appetite, diarrhea or constipation, thick coating on the tongue

- Use the powder of *byi tsher* (cocklebur), *tig ta* (chiretta), *gser gyi me tog* (bolenggua), *bong nga dkar po* (white aconite), *li ga dur* (cranesbill), *dug mo nyung* (kurchi), and *ka ra* (white rock sugar).
- This decoction can also be given: *lcum rtsa* (rhubarb), *dur byid* (spurge), and *a ru ra* (chebulic myrobalan), or the same herbs can be given in powder form, since they are purgative.

Warming or nourishing diets, sudorific therapy, and moxibustion are contraindicated.

Solid Organs Affected by Epidemic Fever

Signs and symptoms: pulse and urine indicative of a hot condition, dry tongue, nonsensical talk, thirst

One of the following three herbs should be selected based on the intensity of the fever: *ga bur* (camphor) for high fever, *tsan dan dkar po* (white sandalwood) for middling fever, or *gi waM* (elephant or ox gallstone) for low-grade fever. This should be mixed with the powder of *cu gang* (bamboo pith), *gur gum* (safflower), *li shi* (clove), *li ga dur* (cranesbill), *tig ta* (chiretta), *bong nga dkar po* (white aconite), *hong len* (picrorhiza grass), and *ka ra* (white rock sugar). Based on the predominance of wind, bile, phlegm, or blood in the disease pattern, the doctor should select from available therapies such as moxibustion, purgation, sudorific therapy, or bloodletting.

Giving nourishing treatment too soon may increase the fever.

Bones Affected by Epidemic Fever

Signs and symptoms: dry nostrils, mouth, and tongue; empty pulse; hearing loss; apathy

Since the wind humor resides in the bones, nourishing treatment, bone soup, etc. are indicated but must be given along with cooling medicines in order to reduce the fever. Moxibustion should be performed on the sixth and seventh vertebrae (T5 and T6).

Cooling the fever without giving nourishment will consume the seven bodily constituents and increase wind.

Treatment Based on the Stage of Illness

It is also possible to stage epidemic fever in phases reminiscent of the three humors. Thus the disease can be seen as progressing from a phlegm-like condition to bile, blood, and wind and blood together, to end as a borderline heat-and-cold disorder. If the disease does not develop according to this pattern during the first eight or nine days, the patient's life may be at risk. The successive stages are described in detail in the rest of this section.

Phlegm Stage

This stage usually corresponds to the first three days of illness. It is also called the phlegm-and-wind stage. Signs and symptoms are headache, pain in the muscles and joints, cold shivering, yawning, apathy, inability to take food (vomiting), and a desire to stay warm. This stage resembles either unripe fever or hidden fever. The fever should be ripened.

A lukewarm decoction of *a ru ra* (chebulic myrobalan), *ba ru ra* (beleric myrobalan), *skyu ru ra* (amla), *ma nu pa tra* (elecampane), *kaNDa ka ri* (two-flowered raspberry), *sle tres* (moonseed), *sga skya* (galangal), *byi tsher* (cocklebur), and *tig ta* (chiretta) should be given to the patient in order to induce sweating, and appropriate dietary and lifestyle recommendations should be observed: as with unripe fever, the food and lifestyle should be warming until the fever ripens into the next stage.

Bile Stage

This stage usually takes place from the fourth to sixth days of illness; it is associated with the bile humor. The sense organs are affected. Signs and symptoms: bitter taste in the mouth, thick coating on the tongue, encrusted lips, dry nostrils, hearing loss, tearing, reddish urine, and tight pulse. This stage is said to resemble a dry river because of the drying effect on the body.

- The patient should be given a cold decoction of *tig ta* (chiretta), *gser gyi me tog* (bolenggua), and *a ru ra* (chebulic myrobalan).
- The patient should also take the powder of *cu gang* (bamboo pith), *gur gum* (safflower), *li shi* (clove), *dzA ti* (nutmeg), *sug smel* (green cardamom), *ka ko la* (black cardamom), *gser gyi me tog* (bolenggua), *ba sha ka* (Malabar nut tree), *li ga dur* (cranesbill), and *ka ra* (white rock sugar). This formula and the one above could be given one after the other or by alternating them morning and evening, depending on the patient's condition.
- If there is headache, the *dpral rtsa* point (at the eyebrows) should be bled, and cool water should be sprinkled at the vertex. (Tibetans believe that the head should be kept cool in order to prevent hair loss.)

Blood Stage

From the seventh to ninth days of illness, the fever affects the blood. The signs and symptoms show more obvious signs of heat, as in the pulse and urine, a dry tongue, thirst, sweating with a strong smell, and a sensation of heaviness. At this stage the fever should be attacked by way of medication the way one attacks an enemy.

The patient should be given the powder of *ga bur* (camphor), *tsan dan dmar po* (red sandalwood), *gi waM* (elephant or ox gallstone), *cu gang* (bamboo pith), *gur gum* (safflower), *li shi* (clove), *li ga dur* (cranesbill), and *ka ra* (white rock sugar). This should be taken consistently every day.

If the blood and/or bile are strongly affected, appropriate purgation and blood-letting therapies should be selected. If there is drowsiness, sudorific therapy should be given, along with cooling diet and lifestyle recommendations.

Wind–and–Blood Stage

Between the tenth and twelfth days from the onset of the disease, both the wind humor and the blood are disturbed, and the solid organs are affected. Signs and symptoms include delirious speech, confusion, loss of consciousness, weakness, submerged pulse, darkened face, and a dry and rough tongue. Treating the patient too aggressively can injure the blood vessels. The treatment should therefore be gentle and use mildly cold medicines.

- The following powder should be taken every morning: *dzA ti* (nutmeg), *snying zho sha* (lapsi tree), *sgog thal* (calcined garlic), and *bur dkar* (white raw cane sugar).
- At the same time, the following powder should be taken mixed with cold water every evening: *ga bur* (camphor), *cu gang* (bamboo pith), and *bong nga dkar po* (white aconite). If there is disturbed fever, substitute *bong nga dkar po* (white aconite) with *tsan dan dmar po* (red sandalwood). This mixture is said to strike high fever like a meteor.

If the life channel is affected, there may be symptoms such as mental disturbance, fighting for no reason, memory loss, impaired speech, bulging eyes, etc. In this case the patient should be given medicinal wine made with *ga bur* (camphor) and *cu gang* (bamboo pith), and the appropriate moxibustion treatment should be given. Garlic water may be helpful. The diet should be warming in the afternoon and cooling in the evening. If the symptoms are not very severe, bloodletting may be effective.

Borderline Heat and Cold Stage

In the three subsequent days, the disease is a borderline hot and cold condition. The wind humor is predominant and the bones are affected. Signs and symptoms are pain in the hips and other bones, weakness, paleness, mental fogginess, tinnitus, and profuse sweating. Diagnosis can be confirmed by tentatively treating the patient with fresh wine in moderate amounts, well-cooked mutton, *bu ram* (raw cane sugar), yogurt, and ankle broth. The treatment approach should be very gentle and consistent with treatment of the wind humor.

If the above diet is helpful, it may be continued and supplemented with the powder of *skyu ru ra* (amla), *tsan dan dkar po* (white sandalwood), *ga bur* (camphor), *sgog thal* (calcined garlic), and *ka ra* (white rock sugar). This powder removes any residual heat.

Treatment of Complex Epidemic Fever

When multiple humors are affected, a general treatment can be applied or the disease can be staged based on the time elapsed since the onset or based on the degree of penetration of the fever.

General Treatment

The general treatment is the decoction of *pa to la* (hyacinth orchid), *pu shel rtse* (noble dendrobium), *gla sgang* (bistort), *shing mngar* (licorice), and *a ru ra* (chebulic myrobalan). This treatment can be applied to any of the first five stages described below.

If the above treatment is not helpful, it may be beneficial to bleed the hand points, except for "one-day fever." One must be careful when reaching the borderline point between heat and cold.

Fever Entering the Nutritive Fluids *(rgun rim)*

This stage represents the fever entering the nutritive fluids. Signs and symptoms suggest the combined involvement of the bile and phlegm humors.

The foundation formula is the decoction of *pa to la* (hyacinth orchid), *dug mo nyung* (kurchi), and *hong len* (picrorhiza grass).

- If there is mostly phlegm, as indicated by belching, vomiting, indigestion, or poor appetite, give the main treatment and add *so cha* (hummingbird tree) and *rgyam tshwa* (rock salt) as emetics.
- If there is mostly bile, as indicated by yellow watery eyes, etc., give the following purgative herbs separately from the main treatment: *dur byid* (spurge), *rgun 'brum* (raisin), *dug mo nyung* (kurchi), *bong nga dkar po* (white aconite), *li ga dur* (cranesbill), and *ba le ka* (birthwort).
- If there is stomach pain caused by microorganisms, give a pill made of *go bye* (marking nut) and *bu ram* (raw cane sugar) in addition to the main formula.

Fever Entering the Blood *(rtag pa'i rim)*

This stage represents the fever entering the blood. Signs and symptoms are pain in the shoulders, stomach or liver discomfort, nosebleed, cough, thick sputum, red and watery eyes, fever, and headache occurring twice a day.

For this condition, give the powder of *hong len* (picrorhiza grass), *pa to la* (hyacinth orchid), *gla sgang* (bistort), *ba spru* (Himalayan mirabilis), and *ma nu pa tra* (elecampane). It may be beneficial to bleed the points that correspond to the most affected area.

One-Day Fever

At this stage the muscles are affected. Signs and symptoms are profuse sweating, sensations of heat and heaviness, mental dullness, and fever.

Give a decoction of *gla sgang* (bistort), *pa to la* (hyacinth orchid), *a ru ra* (chebulic myrobalan), *ba ru ra* (beleric myrobalan), *skyu ru ra* (amla), *nim pa* (neem tree), *dug mo nyung* (kurchi), and *rgun 'brum* (raisin) to bring sweat out, then sprinkle water over the patient's body.

Three-Day Fever

At this stage the fat is affected. Symptoms are drowsiness and mental dullness. Typically there will be a recurring pattern of two days with symptoms and one day without.

- First, give a decoction of *bca' sga* (fresh ginger), *tsan dan dkar po* (white sandalwood), *tig ta* (chiretta), and *sle tres* (moonseed).
- Then give a powder of *byi rug* (*Elsholtzia sp.*), *spos dkar* (frankincense), *yung ba* (turmeric), *skyer pa* (barberry), *brag zhun* (mineral pitch), *dug mo nyung* (kurchi), *bong nga dkar po* (white aconite), *a ru ra* (chebulic myrobalan), *ba ru ra* (beleric myrobalan), and *skyu ru ra* (amla) mixed into a paste with *sbrang rtsi* (honey).

Four-Day Fever

At this stage the bones are affected, and there will be leg pain, joint pain, and pain in the lower back.

- Give a decoction of *sle tres* (moonseed), *gla sgang* (bistort), and *skyu ru ra* (amla).
- Then apply *sle tres* (moonseed) and *brag zhun* (mineral pitch) to the body and rinse with a decoction of *mkhan pa a krong* (*Ajania sp.*).
- Then administer an enema of *ru rta* (costus) and *a ru ra* (chebulic myrobalan) decocted in milk.
- Moxibustion can then be applied to whatever vertebrae feel hollow (give way) and are tender on palpation.

Epidemic Fever Affecting the Brain

This disease pattern probably corresponds to meningitis. In practice the patient is referred to a Western medical facility, and traditional treatment is supportive or complementary. When the patient has recovered, medicinal butter based on the Five Roots and Three Fruits is recommended.

Treatment of Life-Threatening Epidemic Fever

For the most part this section of the Oral Instruction Tantra chapter on epidemic fever is not applicable in contemporary practice. In summary, the headings of this section comprise descriptions and treatments for fever affecting the channels, blood vessels, the head, the lungs, the kidneys, the stomach, and the intestines. There is also a recommended follow-up treatment for residual epidemic fever and a summary of treatment approaches to life-threatening epidemic fever.

Residual Epidemic Fever

If the patient shows signs and symptoms of heat, the treatment of the fever has not been successful. It is then time to give purgatives. After giving purgatives, the stools, urine, and sclera appear yellow for a while, then clear. It is time to stop purgation. The following treatment can then be beneficial:

The patient should be given the powder of *gi waM* (elephant or ox gallstone), *gur gum* (safflower), *dug mo nyung* (kurchi), *hong len* (picrorhiza grass), *tig ta* (chiretta), *skyer pa'i bar shun* (barberry root middle bark), *bong nga dkar po* (white aconite), *kyi lce* (broad-leaf gentian), *gu gul* (myrrh), *lcum rtsa* (rhubarb), and *sgro puShpa*. This powder, to be taken four times a day, will cure residual fever. The patient should not take pungent or light foods, which could harm the life channel; *ga bur* (camphor) is likewise contraindicated.

If the fever persists, the patient should refrain from sweets and dairy products. Bloodletting therapy is contraindicated. The patient should take rice noodles, soup made with popped rice, or water boiled with a little *tsam pa* (roasted barley flour).

Conclusion and Summary

At first, the fever is unripe, so it should be treated with care. When the fever is more developed, it should be brought down more forcefully. At the end of the illness, the body is depleted, and treatment should therefore be applied gently, as if treating an elderly patient.

CRITICAL DIFFERENTIATION BETWEEN HOT AND COLD DISORDERS

The differentiation between heat and cold lies at the heart of any effective therapy. Patients may exhibit superficial signs of cold when they are in fact suffering from hot conditions. Conversely, a patient may present signs of heat and really have a cold illness. Consequently, the doctor must pay close attention to all available signs, symptoms, and other diagnostic criteria, and also be aware of potential sources of error.

Distinguishing Hot and Cold Disorders

Symptoms of a Hot Disorder

- Primary and secondary causes prior to the illness are consistent with those that lead to a hot disease, such as a diet rich in pungent, sharp, and oily foods; anger; overexertion; etc.
- The disease manifests in a dry and hot environment.
- The disease manifests in the dry part of the summer.
- The patient is between ten and forty years of age.
- The patient is primarily of bile constitution.
- The disease affects the parts of the body where the bile resides.
- The symptoms are aggravated at noon and at midnight.
- The symptoms are aggravated during digestion.
- The condition is worsened by taking foods that are hot in nature.
- The urine is reddish, thick, and strong smelling with a lot of fume and sediment.

In addition, one should consider signs that indicate an increase in the bile humor, such as yellow stools and urine, yellow sclera and skin, excessive thirst, a bitter taste in the mouth, headache, and fever.

False Cold and True Heat

Even though a disease may be manifesting the symptoms above, it may also give misleading signs that could be interpreted as signs of cold, such as:

- Signs of phlegm, including mental and physical inertia, poor digestion, poor appetite, stickiness in the mouth with lack of taste, abdominal and lumbar

106

discomfort, loosening of the joints, sunken imperceptible pulse, white and turbid urine with small bubbles, and a pale and moist tongue.

- Signs of wind, such as yawning, insomnia, dizziness, ringing in the ears, moving pains, shivering, joint pain, mental instability, cough with fluid mucus at dawn and in the evening, irregular and floating pulse, bluish urine with large bubbles and no odor or sediment, and a reddish tongue with small pimples.

Such a disease could be a hot condition hidden amidst signs of cold, like embers burning beneath ashes.

Symptoms of a Cold Disorder

- Primary and secondary causes prior to the illness are consistent with those that lead to wind disease, such as a diet rich in bitter, light, and rough foods, exhaustion from excessive sexual intercourse, fasting, insomnia, overexertion on an empty stomach; or causes that would lead to phlegm disease, such as sweet, heavy, cold, and oily foods, lack of activity after meals, being exposed to a cold or damp environment, etc.
- The disease manifests in a cold, windy, or damp environment.
- The disease manifests in the rainy part of the winter.
- The patient is over fifty or a child.
- The patient is primarily of wind or phlegm constitution.
- The disease affects the parts of the body where wind or phlegm reside.
- The symptoms are aggravated at dawn or in the early morning, late afternoon, or evening.
- The symptoms are aggravated right after meals or after digestion.
- The condition is worsened by taking foods that are cold in nature or not very nourishing.
- The urine is bluish with little odor, fume, or sediment.

In addition, one should consider signs that indicate an increase in the wind and phlegm humors, such as abundant viscous saliva, dry and darkened skin, avoidance of cold, and a submerged or floating, halting pulse.

False Heat and True Cold

Even though a disease may be manifesting the symptoms above, it may also give misleading signs that could be interpreted as signs of heat, such as fixed pain, a bitter taste in the mouth, thirst, yellow or red sclera, fever, fatigue, nausea, a thin, fast, and tight pulse, and a yellow-coated tongue.

Sources of Error

Deceptive Disease Names

Relying merely on the mention of a particular disease, an unskilled physician may confuse a hot condition for a cold one. For example, mention of undigested nutritive essence may suggest a phlegm condition, but this could also involve the liver and correspond to an increase of bile. A dark-phlegm condition, which involves fever in the blood, could be taken erroneously as simple phlegm disease.

Likewise, if a doctor hears of poisoning, he or she could assume a hot condition. However, intoxication due to gems or other minerals are of a cold nature. A wrong diagnosis could certainly lead to the wrong treatment and put the patient's life at risk.

Deceptive Symptoms

The following cold conditions may present with misleading signs and symptoms of heat:

- Wind disorders that disturb the blood, causing symptoms such as a bitter taste in the mouth, a dry tongue, and acute pain from one critical point to another of the wind humor
- Phlegm disorders that cause acute pain in the upper part of the body
- Headache due to bile disturbed by the wind humor
- Indigestion where waste products obstruct the channels and invade the gallbladder, resulting in signs such as yellow eyes
- Void fever manifesting after treating a fever disorder

The following hot conditions may present with misleading signs and symptoms of cold:

- Concealed fever in which the digestion is affected, causing the symptoms of a phlegm disorder
- Concealed fever affecting the kidneys, causing symptoms of a cold disorder
- Concealed fever affecting the heart, causing symptoms of a wind disorder
- Minor illnesses such as a fever manifesting as insomnia or vomiting of blood or bile
- A fever that affects the joints, manifesting as joint pain
- A fever that affects the channels, manifesting as yawning and shivering
- A chronic fever that affects the vital channel and manifests as mental instability
- A fever that affects the liver and manifests as sighing

Misleading Treatment Outcomes

The general approach in Tibetan medicine is to direct half of the effort toward treating the humor affected and the other half toward supporting the other two humors. If the emphasis is on the wrong humor, treatment may prove successful at the beginning but ineffective in the long run. For example, treating hidden fever with mostly hot herbs would at first diminish the cold symptoms but prove detrimental over a period of time. Likewise, if a wind disorder presents with a dry tongue, it may seem to be a hot disorder, and cold therapy would produce short-term results but would not be beneficial in the long term.

Deceptive Impressions of the Patient

The patient may erroneously report improvement or worsening over time based on his or her biases and expectations. The doctor should not take those reports at face value but verify them by monitoring the pulse and the urine regularly.

Conclusion

In order to avoid making an erroneous diagnosis, it is important to carefully consider the signs, symptoms, and patient history. If the verdict is mitigated, this may be because the body is weak, as with children or the elderly. In addition, the efficacy of treatment must be constantly evaluated over a long period of time by checking the patient's pulse and urine, which are considered the most reliable indicators of heat or cold. The patient's reporting of improvement or lack thereof must not be taken at face value. Since even the urine can present misleading signs, the sediment must be carefully examined also. All the areas of possible error are collectively known as dangerous places or battlegrounds, because they can lead to an incorrect treatment and therefore the worsening of the patient's condition. While for students of Tibetan medicine these points are only theoretical, a skilled practitioner constantly bears them in mind and develops clinical experience in that area, at times even relying on more experienced, senior doctors when the need arises.

PART III

Therapeutics

Therapeutic Strategies

General Methods

It is best to treat a humor before it has a chance to spread to other locations, i.e. a humor is best treated while it is still confined to its natural location and during the season it accumulates rather than in the season when it arises. The table below summarizes the parts of the year when humors accumulate and arise, respectively:

Humor	Accumulates	Arises
WIND	May and June	July and August
BILE	July and August	September and October
PHLEGM	January and February	March and April

When the humor is still in the phase of accumulation, it is treated by pacifying means without disturbing the other humors. They are best administered at the time of day when the corresponding humor peaks, such as in the morning for phlegm, midday for bile, and in the evening for wind. More specifically, pacifying medicine should be administered thus:

- For disorders involving phlegm or all three humors combined, medicines should be taken on an empty stomach before breakfast.
- For disorders of the purgative wind, medicines should be taken right before meals.
- For disorders of the fire-like wind, medicines should be taken in the middle of the meal.
- For disorders of the pervasive wind, medicines should be taken right after meals.
- For disorders of the life-sustaining wind, medicines should be taken at meals, between mouthfuls.
- For most illnesses and especially for disorders of the ascending wind, medicines should be taken half an hour after meals.
- For breathing problems, medicines should be taken at any time they are needed.
- Medicines should be mixed with food to stimulate the appetite.

- For hiccups, medicines should be taken both just before and just after meals.
- For disorders of the chest and above, medicines should be taken just before bedtime.

If the humor manifests as an illness, cleansing medicines (emetics and purgatives) should be employed. Treatment should not be discontinued until recovery is complete. When the illness has subsided, treatment should be discontinued, or else another imbalance may arise.

Specific Methods

Disorders Accompanied by Indigestion

When the digestive heat is decreased, nutrition is not absorbed as well, and both the pure and impure parts of nutrients get mixed with the seven bodily constituents and with the three excretions. The treatment consists in giving a decoction such as the Three Fruit Decoction or the Decoction of Seven Precious Ingredients to make the disease manifest and at the same time increasing the digestive heat using such medicines as *se 'bru dwangs ma gnas 'jog* (Pomegranate Sanctuary). Then the appropriate cleansing therapy should be employed depending on the location of the illness: suppositories for wind, purgatives for bile, and emetics for phlegm. This should not be attempted before the disease has manifested fully. Cleansing therapy should be applied only when the disease has become manifest, otherwise harm will result and the disease will persist.

Treating a Single Humor

A disorder caused by the imbalance of a single humor is said to be the result of an incorrect diet or lifestyle. The humor will typically increase but remain confined in its own location, and a disease will manifest only when the entire constellation of predisposing factors (diet, behavior, and season) is present. Disorders of a single humor are activated by wind. Therefore most therapy begins by pacifying the wind humor. This has the effect of ripening or gathering the illness, allowing it to manifest. This is similar to rain falling as soon as the wind has stopped. Purgation or emesis (described in the chapter on phlegm) may then be performed. If the illness is not gathered but instead remains spread in the outer parts of the body (limbs, skin, etc.), then it should be treated by bloodletting and/or using medicines that cleanse the channels.

The chief methods for treating wind disorders are:

- For the lifestyle: staying in warm places, enjoying pleasant company, sleeping well, and staying warm
- For diet: nourishing, heavy, oily, smooth, and warming substances such as *bu ram* (raw cane sugar), ale, aged butter,[17] old meat, bone broth, onion, garlic, etc.
- For medicines: *dzA ti* (nutmeg), *shing kun* (asafetida), and medicinal butter made with the Three Fruits and the Five Roots
- For external therapy: massage with old butter and moxibustion

The chief methods for treating bile disorders are:

- For the lifestyle: staying in cool, shady, and breezy places and being undisturbed
- For diet: fresh butter, fresh meat, cold water, black tea, yogurt, buttermilk of cow or goat, cracked-grain porridge, roasted barley flour, and other foods with cooling properties
- For medicines: *ga bur* (camphor), *tsan dan dkar po* (white sandalwood), or *gi waM* (elephant or ox gallstone), depending on the intensity of the fever; and in general purgation and bitter, astringent, and cooling medicines
- For external therapies: sudorific methods, the application of cold water, bloodletting, and cold fomentation

The chief methods for treating phlegm disorders are:

- For the lifestyle: staying warm by staying in the sun or near fires, wearing warm clothing, mental and physical exertion in dry places, and refraining from excessive sleep
- For diet: mutton, fish, old grain, dumplings made from barley flour, warm water, ginger decoction, and other foods with light, coarse, and warming qualities
- For medicines: salty and pungent decoction that include *se 'bru* (pomegranate), *dwa lis* (rhododendron), various calcined medicinals; and in general medicines with sharp, coarse, light, and warming properties, especially emetics
- For external therapies: warm fomentations and moxibustion

Treating a single humor also requires supporting the other two humors so as not to cause imbalance. Using sweet and salty foods, for instance, may decrease wind;

[17.] Butter ages as a result of bacterial action. The bacterial count rises sharply in the first few days after fresh butter is made, and after two months, the amount of bacteria is actually lower than in fresh butter (Heineman 1921).

the sweet taste may increase phlegm; and the salty taste will increase phlegm. Likewise, pungent and sour foods will decrease phlegm, but the pungent taste will increase wind, and the sour taste will increase bile. Treating bile with sweet and bitter foods will decrease bile, but the sweet taste will increase phlegm, and the bitter taste will increase wind. Typically half of the treatment addresses the diseased humor, and the other half of the treatment must support the other two humors.

Superimposed Disorders

New ailments can become superimposed on existing ailments. The new humor typically invades the natural location of the humor that was imbalanced in the first place. If the new ailment is not very serious, it is best to treat the old humor first. The new humor then can no longer invade the location of the humor that was imbalanced originally. However, if the secondary humor does not abate but becomes stronger instead, it should be the main target for treatment, and then the primary humor will be easily treated.

Disorders that Involve Multiple Humors

Treating disorders of combined humors involves balancing the three humors. For this purpose, *a ru ra* (chebulic myrobalan) and *brag zhun* (mineral pitch) are the best remedies. Then specific ingredients may be added based on the condition:

- For heart disorders, *dzA ti* (nutmeg)
- For lung disorders, *cu gang* (bamboo pith)
- For liver disorders, *kha che gur gum* (saffron)
- For disorders of the life channel, *li shi* (clove)
- For kidney disorders, *sug smel* (green cardamom)
- For spleen disorders, *ka ko la* (black cardamom)
- For stomach disorders, *se 'bru* (pomegranate) and *pi pi ling* (long pepper)
- For bile disorders, *tig ta* (chiretta) and *gser gyi me tog* (bolenggua)
- For wind disorders, *dzA ti* (nutmeg), *sle tres* (moonseed), and bone broth
- For phlegm disorders, *ma nu pa tra* (elecampane), *'u su* (coriander), and *bse yab* (Chinese quince)
- For blood disorders, *ba sha ka* (Malabar nut tree) and *hong len* (picrorhiza grass)
- For lymph *(chu ser)* disorders, *spos dkar* (frankincense), *thal ka rdo rje* (foetid cassia), and *so ma rA dza* (aibika)
- For infectious disorders, *gla rtsi* (musk)
- For diseases caused by elemental provocations, *gu gul* (myrrh)

If several conditions occur together, the corresponding respective ingredients should be combined. In addition, the following should be considered when treating multiple humors:

- Treating a combined wind and bile disorder relies on foods and medicines that have cool and nutritious properties.
- Treating a combined phlegm and bile disorder relies on foods and medicines that have cool and light properties.
- Treating a combined wind and phlegm disorder relies on foods and medicines that have warm and nutritious properties.
- Treating a disorder that involves all three humors relies on foods and medicines that have cool, nutritious, and light properties.

Treating multiple humors is likened to being a chieftain who settles a dispute among kinsmen by reducing the humor that is in excess and supporting the humor that is deficient.

If the Diagnosis Is Not Clear

If the diagnosis cannot be formulated clearly, the doctor should proceed "like a cat waiting in ambush." Exploratory treatment should be given for clarity. If the patient improves with a given preliminary treatment, this gives a more solid indication about the nature of the disorder. Examples of exploratory treatments are given below:

- For wind imbalance, bone broth
- For bile, a decoction of *tig ta* (chiretta)
- For phlegm, a decoction of *rgyam tshwa* (rock salt), *sman sga* (ginger), and *a ru ra* (chebulic myrobalan)
- For intestinal infection or parasites, and for stomach or colon disorders, the formula *khyung 5* (Garuda Five)
- For disturbed blood *(khrag 'khrug pa)* or sharp pain caused by wind, the formula Elecampane Four: *ma nu pa tra* (elecampane), *kaNDa ka ri* (two-flowered raspberry), *sle tres* (moonseed), and *sga skya* (galangal)
- For compounded poisons, decoctions that gather the disease
- If heat and cold are intermingled, diet and behavior that promote either heat or cold, based on one's experience

The doctor may also give exploratory treatment in order to predict the efficacy of the therapy being considered, for example:

- A mild purgative to foresee the efficacy of purgation
- Warm oil poultices to foresee the efficacy of moxibustion
- Application of cold water or cold stones on the body to foresee the efficacy of bloodletting

If the Diagnosis Is Firm

If the diagnosis is clear as to the hot or cold nature of the disease, its causative factors and its location in the body, the doctor should proceed to devise an adequate treatment and make a prognosis for recovery (or lack thereof), with the same assurance as if hoisting a banner onto a house or mountaintop.

If the Illness Does Not Respond to Treatment

If the patient does not respond to treatment, one should retrace the steps of the disease carefully. Treatment often fails because of not having separated or gathered the disease properly. For example, treating a fever with cold ingredients if it has not been made fully manifest could result in a combined wind and phlegm imbalance. In this case, the formula Elecampane Four could be used to isolate the culprits wind and phlegm, followed by the treatment of fever.

Likewise, the treatment of blood disorders must be preceded by a decoction of the Three Fruits to separate the pure blood from the impure blood. Only then can bloodletting be performed if required. Performing bloodletting without separating the pure from the impure drains the pure blood and depletes the seven bodily constituents.

Dark phlegm and toxic fevers must likewise be treated by first gathering the illness. Attempting treatment without this preliminary step will spread the disease throughout the body and make it harder to treat.

Hidden fever must be treated first by treating the cold symptoms using warm therapies. Attempting to treat the fever directly with cooling methods exacerbates the cold component of the illness and fails to cool the fever.

Disorders that result in lack of assimilation of nutrients must be treated first by increasing the digestive heat so as to create conditions favorable to recovery. Only when there begin to be signs of improvement can cleansing therapy begin.

If Treatment with another Doctor Was Unsuccessful

If a patient did not respond to treatment given by another doctor, it is necessary to understand whether treatment was excessive, insufficient, or incorrect. Then the doctor can proceed with assurance, like a kingfisher diving into a body of water and coming out with a fish.

Very Serious Disorders

Very serious hot disorders are to be treated with the "four waters": cold medicine (camphor), cold external therapy (bloodletting), a cold diet (light eating or fasting), and a cold lifestyle (staying in cool places). Very serious cold disorders must be treated with the "four fires": hot medicines, hot external therapy (moxibustion), hot (warming and nutritious) diet, and a warming lifestyle (staying in warm places). Since the illness is very serious, all four remedies must be applied at once. Failure to do so is like not using one's weapons when facing an enemy in a narrow pass, and thus may result in death.

Mild Conditions

Mild conditions should be treated progressively, like scaling a ladder one rung at a time. At first, changes in the patient's lifestyle should be tried. If the condition does not improve, dietary changes should be suggested. Then hot or cold medicines should be employed, and only if all the above methods fail should external therapies be given.

Invigoration

Invigoration can be beneficial when there is an excess of wind, depletion of the bodily constituents, depletion caused by excessive sexual intercourse, pregnancy, blood loss (including after giving birth), tuberculosis, old age, insomnia, grief, asceticism, and exhaustion from overwork. It is best undertaken in the dry summer season.

Diet should be nourishing and include mutton, *bu ram* (raw cane sugar), *ka ra* (white rock sugar), butter, milk, yogurt, ale (except of course during pregnancy), etc. The lifestyle should include good sleep, relaxation, and keeping a happy state of mind. Appropriate medicines should be given in the form of medicinal butter. External therapies include enemas, hot springs, medicated steam baths, and massage.

Excessive invigoration leads to obesity, tumors, mental dullness, diabetes, and phlegm. In order to counteract the results of such excessive treatment, foods and medicines with rough qualities should be given, and in particular the following remedies:

- *gu gul* (myrrh), *brag zhun* (mineral pitch), extract of *star bu* (sea buckthorn), and *sbrang rtsi* (honey) dissolved in water

- A decoction of *a ru ra* (chebulic myrobalan), *ba ru ra* (beleric myrobalan), *skyu ru ra* (amla), and *sbrang rtsi* (honey)
- A bolus made of *sman sga* (ginger), *ya bakSha ra* (saltpeter), *byi tang ga* (false black pepper), *skyu ru ra* (amla), barley flour, and *sbrang rtsi* (honey)

In general, it is better to be thin than overweight. Such invigoration therapy should therefore be applied with moderation.

Weight Loss and Fasting

Fasting is desirable if the patient does not assimilate foods, takes excessive amounts of oily and rich foods, or suffers from stiffness due to wind, infectious fever, frequent urination, tumors, arthritis, spleen disorders, throat disorders, brain disorders, heart disorders, fever causing diarrhea or vomiting, lethargy, poor appetite, constipation, urinary retention, obesity, lymph *(chu ser)* disorders, or combined bile and phlegm disorders, and has a surplus of vigor. Fasting is most beneficial in winter. It is contraindicated if the patient is weak or emaciated. Such a patient should receive a mild cleansing treatment instead.

The patient should fast for a sustainable period of time (three days), and then begin eating light, easily digested foods. A patient with moderate strength should then take medicines in powder form to increase digestive heat. A strong patient should undertake physical exercise and use other methods to induce perspiration. The strong patient then requires external therapies such as moxibustion, plasters, fomentation, or bloodletting as indicated. Then cleansing therapy may be initiated depending on the location of the illness:

- If the illness is in the stomach or in the upper part of the small intestine, emesis (described in the chapter on phlegm) should be used.
- If the illness is in the lower part of the small intestine or in the large intestine, an enema should be given.
- If the internal organs are affected, purgation is the method of choice.
- If the disease is scattered throughout the channels, medicines that cleanse the channels should be given.

Fasting clears and sharpens the senses, gives lightness to the body, stimulates the appetite, gives energy and vigor, regulates hunger and thirst, and regularizes the bowels. If performed excessively, it can lead to emaciation, dizziness, insomnia, a dull complexion, thirst, anorexia, various aches, nausea, and a propensity to wind disorders, colds, and influenza. In order to restore the depletion caused by excessive fasting, the patient should be given invigorating treatment as described above.

Summary

In performing diagnosis, the doctor must bear these ten points in mind:

1. The state of the patient's seven bodily constituents and three excretions
2. The climate where the patient lives
3. The season when the disease becomes manifest
4. The patient's constitutional type
5. The patient's age
6. The humor at the origin of the disorder
7. The location of the illness
8. The state of the patient's digestive heat
9. The patient's energy level and its changes through various circumstances
10. The patient's readiness to make lifestyle and dietary changes toward the betterment of his or her health

If all the above factors are consistent with one another, then therapy may be applied forcefully. If they are inconsistent, the doctor should retain the criteria that provide the clearest indication and proceed with treatment in a measured way, in proportion to the severity of the disease.

LIFESTYLE

One should be mindful of one's lifestyle in order to preserve and prolong life. The most obvious recommendation is to avoid risks such as drowning, attacks, falls, robbery, landslides, earthquakes, etc.

One's sleep should be sufficient to ensure rest. Not sleeping at night stirs up the wind humor. Likewise, sleeping during the day causes phlegm to arise. However, people suffering from the wind humor can benefit from extra rest during the day when the days are longer (May or June) and the season manifests a rough energy. If sleep is lost during the night, it is recommended to sleep again for half of the time missed just before breakfast. Insomnia can be remedied by taking hot milk, meat broth, or alcohol. Massage with sesame oil, especially over the head, and pouring a bit of sesame oil into the ears can also help. Excessive sleep can be remedied by taking emetics, fasting, stimulating conversation, and sexual intercourse.

Unsafe sexual behavior, adultery, and intercourse during menstruation or pregnancy should be avoided. Weak, unpleasant, and very unhappy partners should be avoided. In winter, there is no restriction on the amount of intercourse. In spring and autumn, this activity should be limited to ten times per month. In summer, when sexual energy is at its lowest, it should be limited to twice a month.

Massage (which in Tibetan medicine involves the application of oil) is very beneficial in preventing wind disorders. One should not overexert oneself immediately after massage. However, in winter and spring, persons of phlegm constitution can perform heavier physical activity after massage.

Natural medicinal baths (hot springs) of different kinds are described in the chapter on hot disorders. They have numerous benefits, including enhancing sexual potency, promoting bodily heat, increasing vigor, etc. The head should not be bathed for it is said that this will cause hair loss and harm to the eyes. Medicinal baths are contraindicated for hot diarrhea, abdominal distention, colds, digestive problems, eye disorders, and ear disorders. One should also not take a medicinal bath right after a meal.

The eyes should be well looked after, since they are one of the most important organs. As a preventive measure, it is possible to wash the eyes once a week with concentrated extract of *skyer pa* (barberry).

Advice is also given to practice sound worldly ways and ethics. This entails keeping one's promises, thinking before speaking or acting, not being swayed by what people say, being of stable character, being loyal, living in harmony with others, refraining from envy or pride based on one's wealth or social status, etc.

Spiritual (i.e. Buddhist) ethics are also advised, namely refraining from killing, stealing, sexual misconduct, improper speech (lying, idle chatter, harsh speech, and divisive gossip), and improper thoughts (covetousness, malice, and wrong views[18]). Furthermore, one should engage in deeds that benefit others, and cherish all living beings, understanding that like us, all wish to be happy and avoid suffering.

Seasonal behavior deals with adjusting one's lifestyle and diet to suit the season. In winter, the body's digestive bile surges and can easily harm the blood and other bodily constituents. One should therefore eat more sweet, sour, and salty foods to counterbalance the upsurge of digestive heat. One should also stay warm and eat rich foods such as meat, raw cane sugar, bone broth, and alcohol.[19]

In the spring, phlegm increases and can weaken the digestive heat. One should therefore eat more bitter, pungent, and astringent foods, do some exercise, and reduce phlegm by other means.

In the first (dry) part of the summer, the body is weaker and must therefore be replenished with sweet, dry, oily, and cool properties. One should wear light clothing, stay in well-ventilated areas, avoid salty, sour, and pungent foods, take medicines that pacify wind, refrain from exercise, and not stay in the sun too long.

In the second (humid) part of the summer, the digestive heat is weakened. One should take medicines that strengthen the digestive heat, eat sweet, sour, and salty foods that have light, oily, and warming properties, and stay away from dampness.

In the fall, the bile humor is stronger, and one should therefore eat more sweet, bitter, and astringent foods and take purgative medicines.

One should allow natural bodily functions such as hunger, thirst, vomiting, sneezing, yawning, breathing, sleeping, expectoration, lacrimation, defecation, flatulence, urination, and seminal emission. Various disorders arise when any of the above is suppressed rather than allowed to occur.

[18.] Wrong views are those philosophical and religious stances that are incompatible with the Buddhist doctrine of egolessness and must therefore be avoided as not conducive to enlightenment. They fall into the two categories of eternalism (the belief that the soul exists forever) and nihilism (the belief that all of one's self, including one's karma, disappears at the moment of death). For more details see the *Brahmajāla Sutta* (Walshe 1987).

[19.] While alcohol is a source of calories, one could argue that it also increases peripheral circulation and therefore creates a warm sensation while at the same time increasing the loss of bodily heat.

Diet

As part of the consultation, the practitioner will typically recommend some foods to be preferred and others to be avoided. This follows a logic similar to that of prescribing herbs, namely based on the taste, post-digestive taste, and intrinsic properties of foods, as described in detail in Chapters 19 and 20 of the Explanatory (Second) Tantra. Below are lists of common foods with their properties and actions, adapted from a more complete work on the vegetal foodstuffs used in Tibetan medicine (Men-Tsee-Khang 2006) and from other sources.

Properties of Common Foods

Meats

- Beef is cold and oily and treats fever associated with wind.
- Crab treats urinary retention.
- Fish is warming, treats digestive problems, stimulates the appetite, benefits the eyes, heals ulcers and wounds, treats phlegm, and reduces certain kinds of tumors.
- Mutton is oily and warming, increases vigor and the bodily constituents, treats wind and phlegm, and stimulates the appetite.
- Pork is cold and light, heals inflammation caused by ulcers and wounds, and treats dark phlegm.
- Poultry is warming, boosts reproductive fluids and bodily constituents, and heals ulcers and wounds.

Grains and Seeds

- Barley is sweet, heavy, and cold, increases the volume of feces, and increases physical vigor.
- Corn (maize) is sweet, astringent, and cooling and relieves bile fever, inflammation, leukorrhea, water retention, poisoning, and constipation but can worsen phlegm somewhat.
- Flax seed is sweet, bitter, and warming and pacifies wind but can worsen indigestion and bile.
- Peanut is sweet and warm, nourishes the bodily constituents, increases sexual potency, pacifies wind, and benefits the skin and channels but is contraindicated for heart disorders, hypertension, and high blood cholesterol.

- Rice is sweet, oily, smooth, cooling, and light, balances the three humors, increases virility, and stops diarrhea and vomiting.
- Sesame seed is sweet and warming, treats wind disorders, increases the digestive heat, nourishes the bodily constituents, helps sleep, treats impotence, benefits the skin, and promotes the growth of hair but can worsen fever and combined bile and phlegm disorders.
- Soybean is sweet and neutral, increases bodily constituents, pacifies wind, is diuretic, reduces swelling, and neutralizes poisons.
- Sunflower seed is sweet and warming, nourishes the kidneys and the bodily constituents, relieves phlegm and cough, and treats wind and swelling during pregnancy but can worsen bile and fever disorders.
- Wheat is sweet, heavy, and cold, increases physical vigor, and pacifies wind and bile disorders.

Fruits and Vegetables

- Asparagus is sweet and neutral, nourishes the blood and semen, strengthens the body, removes water, phlegm, and lymph (chu ser) and is beneficial for diabetes, fatigue, and impotence but can be harmful in cases of diarrhea, urinary infection, gout, and swelling of the feet.
- Aubergine: see eggplant.
- Bamboo shoot is sweet, slightly sour, and cooling, helps heal wounds, treats lung fever, chronic fever, thirst caused by stomach heat, and inflammation, and helps prevent cancer and constipation but is not recommended in cases of weak digestion.
- Beet (beetroot) is sweet and cooling, nourishes the blood, reduces bile fever, poisoning, and dysentery, and benefits the skin but can worsen cold digestive disorders.
- Beetroot: see beet.
- Bitter melon (bitter gourd) is bitter and cooling, alleviates many hot disorders, and is particularly beneficial for diabetes but is not advised for patients with a weak digestive system or stomach disorders.
- Broccoli is sweet, salty, and slightly cooling, increases the blood and bodily constituents, treats inflammation, increases digestive heat, and helps prevent diabetes and cancer but can increase phlegm and cold.
- Cabbage (red or green) is sweet and cooling, helps digestive disorders, helps sleep, and helps prevent wind-related heart disorders and cancer but can aggravate phlegm and cold. It can be applied externally for various skin disorders.

- Carrot is sweet and neutral, nourishes the blood and the liver, benefits the eyes, and helps prevent cancer but can worsen weakened digestion.
- Cauliflower is sweet and slightly cooling, helps nourish the blood and other bodily constituents, reduces inflammation, pacifies wind, and helps prevent cancer but can worsen phlegm, gout, and arthritis.
- Courgette: see zucchini.
- Cucumber is sweet, astringent, and cooling, relieves fever, thirst, and water retention, and treats hot diarrhea but can worsen weakened digestion and cold diarrhea. Applied externally, it benefits the skin and treats burns.
- Eggplant (aubergine) is sweet and slightly cooling. It treats heat and blood disorders but can worsen weakened digestion and chronic diarrhea.
- French bean: see green bean.
- Green bean (French bean) is sweet, astringent, neutral, and oily, pacifies wind, and increases vitality but can worsen bile and phlegm.
- Lady's finger: see okra.
- Leek is pungent, sweet, and warming, improves digestion, helps sleep, and relieves wind but can increase bile.
- Lettuce is sweet, bitter, and slightly cooling, benefits the channels and the blood, regulates the bowels, and promotes lactation.
- Lotus root is sweet, astringent, and neutral, nourishes the bodily constituents, helps sleep, and cools fever but can be harmful to a weak digestive system.
- Mushrooms in general are sweet, salty, and neutral, neutralize poisons, and heal wounds but worsen phlegm and gout.
- Okra (lady's finger) is astringent, sweet, and cooling, treats inflammation of the kidneys and bladder, relieves fever and water retention, smoothens and brightens the skin, and treats diarrhea and impotence but can worsen phlegm and cold conditions.
- Onion is warming, helps sleep, stimulates the appetite, and treats phlegm and wind disorders.
- Pea is sweet and cooling, collects toxins, pacifies bile, and improves the appetite but can worsen wind, phlegm, and cold disorders.
- Potato and sweet potato are sweet and cooling, prevent nausea, and relieve gastritis, stomach cramps, and constipation but can be harmful for phlegm disorders or when there is asthma, diabetes, genital disorders, or obesity; this is especially true of sweet potato.
- Radish is sweet, pungent, and warming, helps digestion, and treats wind but can worsen bile and blood disorders.

- Raisin benefits the lungs.
- Sweet potato: see potato.
- Tomato is sour, sweet, and cooling, treats fever and blood disorders, relieves thirst, stops bleeding, helps digestion, and improves vision, but consumed raw it can harm the skin, worsen lymph *(chu ser)* disorders, and cause headache, and taken cooked it can worsen bile and blood disorders.
- Turnip is pungent, sweet, and warming, prevents and treats poisoning, and pacifies wind but can worsen diarrhea and bile disorders.
- Zucchini (courgette) is sweet, bitter, and slightly cooling, nourishes the bodily constituents, and helps lactation.

Spices

- Black pepper treats phlegm and cold disorders and improves the appetite.
- Caraway treats fever associated with wind, fever in the heart and phlegm, and restores digestive heat.
- Chili pepper: see hot pepper.
- Cinnamon treats cold disorders and wind disorders of the liver and stomach, restores digestive heat, and improves digestion.
- Clove treats disorders of the life channel, treats wind, improves digestion and appetite, and restores warmth of the liver and stomach.
- Coriander restores digestive heat, treats phlegm and dark phlegm, and relieves abdominal spasms.
- Cumin increases digestive heat and improves the appetite.
- Fennel is sweet, warming, increases digestive heat, and removes intestinal parasites but can increase bile and menstrual bleeding and is contraindicated during pregnancy.
- Garlic treats wind and wind-related fever, increases digestive heat, and expels parasites.
- Ginger increases the appetite, restores digestive heat, and treats wind and phlegm disorders.
- Green cardamom warms the kidneys, increases digestive heat, and improves physical strength.
- Hot pepper (chili pepper) is warming, increases digestive heat, eases hemorrhoids, lymph *(chu ser)* disorders, dropsy, and leprosy, kills bacteria, and prevents tumors and cysts but can worsen hot and bile conditions, bleeding disorders, lung infections, eye diseases, and stomach problems.
- Nutmeg treats wind disorders and heart disorders and alleviates depression and sadness.

- Saffron is sweet, bitter, and cooling and benefits the liver but can increase cold and phlegm.
- Salt improves digestion and adds flavor to the food.
- Star anise is sweet and warming, relieves cold digestive disorders, and eases kidney pain but can aggravate blood and bile disorders.
- Turmeric treats infectious disorders, removes toxins, and stops tissue necrosis.

Dairy Products

- Cow's milk is sweet, oily, and heavy, increases bodily constituents, enhances the complexion, treats wind and bile, increases reproductive fluids, prevents consumption, chronic infection, and diabetes, sharpens the mind, and alleviates breathing problems. However, its cold and heavy nature increases phlegm. To lessen this heavy quality, milk can be mixed with an equal amount of water and boiled down to half the volume. This makes the milk light and warming (Thubten Phuntsog 2001).
- Yogurt is sour, cold, and oily, stimulates the appetite, and treats constipation and fever associated with wind.

Hot Drinks

- Cocoa is sweet and neutral, strengthens the body, nourishes the blood, and induces urination but can aggravate wind disorders and polyuria.
- Coffee is sweet, bitter, and cooling, increases energy, is diuretic, and improves blood circulation but can aggravate wind disorders.
- Green tea is bitter, sweet, and cooling, relieves fever and thirst, and makes the body lighter but can increase wind.
- Nettle is sweet and warming, helps digestion, and pacifies wind, but can aggravate bile and phlegm disorders.

Sweeteners

- Raw cane sugar benefits wind disorders. Unsulfured blackstrap molasses (treacle) probably has similar or even stronger effects.
- Refined white sugar benefits bile disorders.
- Honey benefits phlegm and lymph (*chu ser*) disorders.

Dietary Habits

The Explanatory (Second) Tantra contains various recommendations concerning foods and food combinations to be avoided, the correct amount of food to be eaten, etc. Notably, it is considered unwholesome to eat while still digesting the previous meal.

The correct amount of food to be taken depends on its digestibility. When eating light foods, the stomach can be filled. When eating heavy foods, only half the stomach should be filled. In general, the stomach should be filled halfway with food and one quarter with drink. The remaining quarter of the stomach should be left open for the digestive processes to take place properly. Overfilling the stomach impairs digestion, deteriorates the digestive heat, and produces phlegm. Not eating enough fails to nourish the body properly and produces wind.

Persons who desire to put on weight should take alcohol. Persons who desire to lose weight should drink honey dissolved in water.

Materia Medica

Introduction

This chapter describes the most commonly used herbs in Tibetan medicine. For brevity the term herb also includes roots, trees, vegetal extracts, animal products, and minerals. The herbs are presented individually in this chapter in order to provide a foundation. In practice they are rarely given singly. The mainstay of Tibetan therapeutics is made up of pills based on time-tested formulas, the most common of which are presented in the next chapter.

Herb Categories

In order to facilitate study, the herbs are grouped into functional categories loosely based on the categories described in the Blue Beryl commentary and in Chapter 21 of the Explanatory (Second) Tantra. The herbs were also classified into categories based on their actual actions and uses. Within each category, the herbs appear in decreasing order of prevalence within this text.

Wylie Transliteration

In this text the Wylie system is used to transliterate Tibetan names into the Roman alphabet. This widely accepted scheme can accurately transcribe the spelling of the Tibetan original, but it does not reflect pronunciation. The reader who wants to know the pronunciation of the names of Tibetan herb needs to study Tibetan orthography, described in many language manuals (Tournadre 2003). A system of extensions to the original Wylie system has been proposed by the Tibetan and Himalayan Digital Library of the University of Virginia to accommodate the transliteration of Tibetan words of Sanskrit origin (Garson and Germano 2004). A summary of the extended Wylie transliteration scheme as it pertains to this book is presented in an appendix.

Drug Names versus Botanical Names

There is an immediate problem translating the Tibetan names of plant ingredients into any language: a Tibetan drug name does not describe a single plant entity but rather a group of plants that may be used for accomplishing a specific therapeutic goal. For example, *tig ta* can be any one of three or more different plants, including *Swertia chirayita, Swertia ciliata,* and *Saxifraga umbellulata.* This work nudges the reader toward the use of *Swertia chirayita* as more commonly available and with better-researched pharmacology, but this choice is not claimed as authoritative. Kletter and Kriechbaum (2001) explain that one of the authors, Dawa, "refers to *tig ta* as a group of plants [that] all have a bitter taste (*tig* means bitter) and are used similarly." Rather than botanical identification, the name *tig ta* means the more abstract principle of a broadly used, bitter herb with cold properties suitable for the general treatment of bile disorders.

In English, a plant's common name can be used to convey a similar idea. A lot of common names are vague in that they often identify a plant genus rather than a single species. Firstly, this approximates the banality and versatility that is often implicit in Tibetan herb names. It is clearly the intention of Tibetan medicine to encourage practitioners to rely on readily-available plant materials wherever they may be found. For example, in this work *khur mang* has been given as dandelion without raising the question of whether it should be the dandelion of Western herbalists *(Taraxacum officinale)*, that of Chinese herbalists *(Taraxacum mongolicum)*, that of Tibet *(Taraxacum tibetanum)*, that of Sikkim *(Taraxacum sikkimense)* or any of a great many other dandelion species. While there is no question that different species of dandelion can have different clinical effects, the substitution is reasonable if the clinician is aware of possible differences. This of course entails extensive knowledge of and clinical experience with the materia medica actually being used.

Furthermore, in many cases the botanical identification is still in question. Using an English common name leaves room for further refining while still conveying a general idea about the plant. Considerable effort has been expended in recouping available information to resolve the many contradictions concerning the exact species. Many such apparent contradictions may in fact be due to local variability. Accordingly, the botanical names given may not be the only suitable species for the drug, nor are they offered as definitive identification. Other authors have spent much more time researching the identification of Tibetan plant drugs and describing the difficulty thereof (Aschoff and Rösing 1997; Clark 2000; Kletter and Kriechbaum 2001).

Some of the plants have no English common name and were given a drug name for convenience. These coinages are:

*   Bolenggua for *gser gyi me tog (Herpetospermum pedunculosum)*, based on a Chinese drug name.[20] *Bo leng gua zi* (波棱瓜子) designates the seed of three possible plants, including the above, all of which have very similar pharmacological properties. Refer to the plant's entry for further discussion.

[20.] Likewise, a Chinese drug name often subsumes several plant species, mainly because of regional variations.

- Broad-leaf gentian for *kyi lce* and small-leaf gentian for *spang rgyan,* each of which is a collective name for a number of gentian species. Tibetans distinguish these two kinds of gentian based on the size of their leaves. This taxonomy is also consistent with the two respective Chinese drug names, *qin jiao* (秦艽) and *long dan cao* (龙胆草). It seems fitting to capture the distinction in English as well.
- Tartar chrysanthemum for *a byag gzer 'joms (Chrysanthemum tatsienense)* is a loose translation of one of the plant's Chinese names: *chuan xi xiao huang ju* (川西小黄菊).
- Lhasa saxifrage for *sum cu tig* is a translation of the Latin name *Saxifraga lhasana.*

False Friends

Some herbs' Tibetan names are clearly of Sanskrit origin but refer to different herbs than the Ayurvedic herbs that bear similar names. The table below illustrates common areas of confusion. For further clarification, refer to the herbs' respective entries and other relevant literature, especially that which includes illustrations or photographs.

Tibetan name	Herb identification	Sanskrit name	Ayurvedic herb	References
kaNDa ka ri	Two-flowered raspberry (*Rubus biflorus*)	*Kantkari*	Yellow-berried nightshade (*Solanum xanthocarpum*)	Chinese Materia Medica 2002; Dawa 2009; Pasang Yonten Arya 1998; Tendzin Dakpa 2007; Tsewang Tsarong 1994
ut pal	Himalayan poppy (*Meconopsis sp.*)	*Utpala*	Water lily (*Nymphaea sp.*)	Chinese Materia Medica 2002; Dawa 2009; Pasang Yonten Arya 1998; Tendzin Dakpa 2007
nA ga ge sar, pad ma ge sar, etc.	Silk cotton tree (*Bombax ceiba*)	*Nagkesar*	Cobra's saffron (*Mesua ferea*)	Chinese Materia Medica 2002; Dawa 2009; Pasang Yonten Arya 1998; Tendzin Dakpa 2007

Herbs That Treat Wind

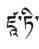

Wylie	*dzA ti*
Drug name	Nutmeg
Botanical name	*Myristica fragrans*
Part used	Seed
Taste and properties	Acrid; oily and heavy

Traditional Actions and Clinical Uses

- Treats wind disorders and heart disorders: this is one of the Six Excellent Drugs used in many formulas.
- Nutmeg may be taken with butter or ale to alleviate depression and sadness (Thubten Phuntsog 2001).

Procurement

Nutmeg is a common spice.

Known Pharmacological Properties

Nutmeg has antidiarrheal, antidotal, amphetamine antagonist, hepatoprotective, hypotensive, hypolipidemic, CNS depressant, diaphoretic, diuretic, psychotropic, smooth-muscle relaxant, prostaglandin-synthetase inhibitor, antioxidant, anti-thrombotic, analgesic, anti-inflammatory, and antitumor actions (Caldecott 2006; Ross 2001).

ལི་ཤི་

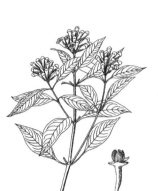

Wylie	*li shi*
Drug name	Clove
Botanical name	*Syzygium aromaticum* syn. *Eugenia caryophyllata*
Part used	Seed
Taste and properties	Acrid; warming and oily

Traditional Actions and Clinical Uses

Treats disorders of the life channel, treats wind, improves digestion and appetite, and restores warmth of the liver and stomach: this is one of the Six Excellent Drugs used in many formulas.

Procurement

Clove is a common spice.

Known Pharmacological Properties

Clove has antibiotic, antiparasitic, gastric stimulant, and uterotonic actions (Bensky and Gamble 1986). Antiulcer action has been reported.

Additional Reference

Al-Mofleh, I. A., A. A. Alhaider, J. S. Mossa, M. O. Al-Sohaibani, S. Qureshi, and S. Rafatullah. 2005. Pharmacological studies on 'clove' *Eugenia caryophyllata. Pharmacognosy Magazine* 1 (3):105–9.

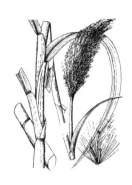

 བུ་རམ་

Wylie	*bu ram*
Drug name	Raw cane sugar
Latin name	*Saccharum officinarum*
Taste and properties	Sweet; warming

Traditional Actions and Clinical Uses

Serves as a vehicle for preparations used to treat wind disorders.

Procurement and Variants

Raw cane sugar is available from Indian grocery stores where it is known as *jaggery* or *jagri*. The best type is white and from sugarcane. The dark sugar-beet variety is considered inferior. Chinese red sugar, known as *hong tang* (红糖), available from Chinese grocery stores, may also be considered (Chinese Materia Medica 2002). Unsulfured blackstrap molasses (treacle) is probably equivalent or better. The common brown sugar sold in supermarkets, being much more refined, is probably very similar to white sugar.

Known Pharmacological Properties

Most research cited here pertains to sugarcane extract, where the sugar itself has been reduced or eliminated. Hepatoprotective, immune-boosting, endurance-enhancing, and hypoglycemic actions have been reported (Ross 2001). Claims of cholesterol-lowering effects have been largely invalidated.

Additional References

Arruzazabala, M. L., D. Carbajal, R. Mas, V. Molina, S. Valdes, and A. Laguna. 1994. Cholesterol-lowering effects of policosanol in rabbits. *Biological Research* 27 (3–4): 205–8.

Carr, T. P., C. L. Weller, V. L. Schlegel, S. L. Cuppett, D. M. Guderian Jr., and K. R. Johnson. 2005. Grain sorghum lipid extract reduces cholesterol absorption and plasma non-HDL cholesterol concentration in hamsters. *Journal of Nutrition* 135 (9): 2236–40.

Francini-Pesenti, F., D. Beltramolli, S. Dall'acqua, and F. Brocadello. 2008. Effect of sugarcane policosanol on lipid profile in primary hypercholesterolemia. *Phytotherapy Research* 22 (3): 318–22.

Greyling, A., C. De Witt, W. Oosthuizen, and J. C. Jerling. 2006. Effects of a policosanol supplement on lymph lipid concentrations in hypercholesterolaemic and heterozygous familial hyper-cholesterolaemic subjects. *British Journal of Nutrition* 95 (5): 968–75.

Holt, S., V. D. Jong, E. Faramus, T. Lang, and J. Brand Miller. 2003. A bioflavonoid in sugarcane can reduce the postprandial glycaemic response to a high-GI starchy food. *Asia Pacific Journal of Clinical Nutrition* 12 (supplement): S66

Kabir, Y., and S. Kimura. 1995. Tissue distribution of (8-14C)-octacosanol in liver and muscle of rats after serial administration, *Annals of Nutrition and Metabolism* 39 (5): 279–8.

Kassis, A. N., S. Kubow, and P. J. Jones. 2009. Sugarcane policosanols do not reduce LDL oxidation in hypercholesterolemic individuals. *Lipids* 44 (5): 391–6.

Keller, S., F. Gimmler, and G. Jahreis. 2008. Octacosanol administration to humans decreases neutral sterol and bile acid concentration in feces. *Lipids* 43 (2): 109–15.

Marinangeli C. P., A. N. Kassis, D. Jain, N. Ebine, S. C. Cunnane, and P. J. Jones. 2007. Comparison of composition and absorption of sugarcane policosanols. *British Journal of Nutrition* 97 (2): 381–8.

Ng, C. H., K.Y. Leung, Y. Huang, and Z. Y. Chen. 2005. Policosanol has no antioxidant activity in human low-density lipoprotein but increases excretion of bile acids in hamsters. *Journal of Agricultural and Food Chemistry* 53 (16): 6289–93.

Nikitin, I. P., N. V. Slepchenko, N. A. Gratsianskiĭ, A. S. Nechaev, A. L. Syrkin, M. G. Poltavskaia, A. V. Sumarokov, and A. V. Revazov. 2000. Results of the multicenter controlled study of the hypolipidemic drug polycosanol in Russia. *Terapevticheskiĭ Arkhiv* (in Russian) 72 (12): 7–10.

Ohta, Y., K. Ohashi, T. Matsura, K. Tokunaga, A. Kitagawa, and K. Yamada. 2008. Octacosanol attenuates disrupted hepatic reactive oxygen species metabolism associated with acute liver injury progression in rats intoxicated with carbon tetrachloride. *Journal of Clinical Biochemistry and Nutrition* 42 (2): 118–25.

Singh, D. K., L. Li, and T. D. Porter. 2006. Policosanol inhibits cholesterol synthesis in hepatoma cells by activation of AMP-kinase. *Journal of Pharmacology and Experimental Therapeutics* 318 (3): 1020–6.

Tedeschi-Reiner, E., Z. Reiner, Z. Romić, and D. Ivanković. 2005. A randomized, double-blind, placebo-controlled study of the antilipemic efficacy and tolerability of food supplement policosanol in patients with moderate hypercholesterolemia. *Liječnički Vjesnik* (in Croatian) 127 (11–12): 273–9.

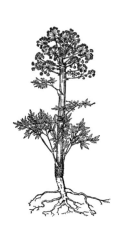

ཤིང་ཀུན་

Wylie	*shing kun*
Drug name	Asafetida
Botanical name	*Ferula asafoetida*
Part used	Resin
Taste and properties	Acrid; warming

Traditional Actions and Clinical Uses

- Treats heart wind conditions.
- Treats cold disorders.
- Expels worms.

Procurement

Asafetida extract can be found at Indian grocery stores (usually mixed with flour), where it is known as *hing*.

Known Pharmacological Properties

Asafetida has antispasmodic, antithrombotic, hypotensive, anti-inflammatory, antiulcer, phosphatase and sucrase inhibiting, smooth-muscle relaxant, vasodilatory, pancreatic amylase and chymotrypsin stimulant, anticonvulsant, antibacterial, aphrodisiac, antioxidant, and anticancer actions (Caldecott 2006; Ross 2005).

ལྩ་བ་

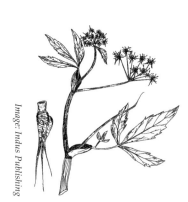

Image: Indus Publishing

Wylie	*lca ba*
Drug name	Angelica
Botanical name	*Angelica glauca*
Part used	Root
Taste and properties	Sweet and acrid; warming and heavy

Traditional Actions and Clinical Uses

- Treats wind disorders: angelica is most often used in combination with *ba spru* (Himalayan mirabilis), *ra mnye* (Solomon's seal), *gze ma* (puncture vine), and *nye shing* (asparagus) for the treatment of wind.
- Removes lymph *(chu ser)* accumulations in the joints.
- Restores kidney heat.
- Treats stomach disorders.

Procurement and Variants

This herb is probably the same as *chorak* or *choraka (Angelica glauca)*, available from Ayurvedic herbalists. It has become threatened in the Indian state of Himachal Pradesh (Badola and Pal 2002). According to its pharmacological properties, there are also similarities with *Angelica archangelica*, available from Western herbalists. See the references below for more details on possible identifications.

Known Pharmacological Properties

Angelica archangelica has diaphoretic, expectorant, estrogenic, analgesic, smooth-muscle relaxant, antiallergic, immunomodulatory, antibacterial, vasodilator, and spasmolytic actions, as well as other beneficial cardiovascular effects (Willard 1991).

Additional References

Committee on Herbal Medicinal Products. 2007. *Reflection paper on the risks associated with furocoumarins contained in preparations of* Angelica archangelica L. London: European Medicines Agency.

Sarker, S. D., and L. Nahar. 2004. Natural medicine: The genus *Angelica. Current Medicinal Chemistry* 11 (11): 1479–1500.

Torkelson, Anthony R. 1999. *The cross name index to medicinal plants: Plants in Indian medicine.* Boca Raton, Fla.: CRC Press.

 རི་བོང་སྙིང་

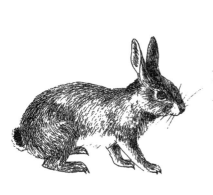

Wylie	*ri bong snying*
Drug name	Hare heart
Latin name	*Lepus sp.*
Part used	Heart
Taste and properties	Sweet

Traditional Actions and Clinical Uses

- Treats diseases caused by the spirit named *skem byed* (*Skanda* in Sanskrit), a demon that causes disease in children.
- Treats wind disorders of the heart and heart pain.

Procurement and Variants

Rabbit is a common meat in many Western countries and a likely substitute for hare.

Reference

Strickmann, Michel, and Bernard Faure. 2002. *Chinese magical medicine.* Palo Alto, Calif.: Stanford University Press.

Herbs That Treat Fever Associated with Wind

 རུ་རྟ་

Wylie	*ru rta*
Drug name	Costus
Botanical name	*Saussurea lappa* syn. *Aucklandia lappa*
Part used	Root
Taste and properties	Acrid and bitter; warm, oily, and sharp

Traditional Actions and Clinical Uses

- Treats wind and blood disorders.
- Restores digestive heat.
- Treats disturbed fever.
- Treats disorders of the life-sustaining wind.
- Because of its action on the blood, costus is also used in the treatment of bile and yellow phlegm.
- Costus directs the action of a formula to the large intestine (Dawa 1999).

Procurement and Variants

Tibetan medicine knows two varieties of costus. The white variety, *ru rta dkar po (Vladimiria souliei)* from Kham is considered superior, but it has become rare. The black variety, *ru rta nag po (Saussurea lappa),* is available from Chinese herbalists as *mu xiang* (木香) and from Ayurvedic herbalists as *kut* or *kustha*. It has become threatened in the Indian state of Himachal Pradesh (Badola and Pal 2002).

Known Pharmacological Properties

Costus has an antiulcer action and can stimulate the motility of the upper gastrointestinal tract. It has bronchodilator, antispasmodic, hypotensive, heart-inhibiting, and antibacterial actions (Bensky and Gamble 1986; Caldecott 2006; Chang and But 1986).

སློ་ཏྲེས་

Wylie	*sle tres*
Drug name	Moonseed
Botanical name	*Tinospora cordifolia*
Part used	Twigs
Taste and properties	Sweet, bitter, astringent, and acrid; cool and oily

Traditional Actions and Clinical Uses

- Treats fever and unripe fever associated with wind: moonseed is often used in combination with *ma nu pa tra* (elecampane), *kaNDa ka ri* (two-flowered raspberry), and *sga skya* (galangal) to treat recently acquired fever, to gather or ripen fever, or to make hidden fever manifest.
- Treats gout and premature aging due to depleted bodily constituents: moonseed is considered one of the best remedies for gout.

Procurement

Moonseed is available from Ayurvedic herbalists as *guruchi.*

Known Pharmacological Properties

Moonseed has anticancer, antioxidant, antistress, antiulcer, immunomodulatory, hepatoprotective, and hypoglycemic actions (Williamson 2002). In human trials, it was shown to have a significant effect on allergic rhinitis (Caldecott 2006).

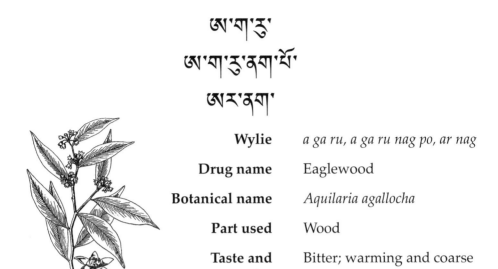

ཨ་ག་རུ་
ཨ་ག་རུ་ནག་པོ་
ཨར་ནག་

Wylie	*a ga ru, a ga ru nag po, ar nag*
Drug name	Eaglewood
Botanical name	*Aquilaria agallocha*
Part used	Wood
Taste and properties	Bitter; warming and coarse

Traditional Actions and Clinical Uses

- Treats fever of the heart and life channel.
- Eaglewood is used to treat disorders of the accomplishing bile.

Procurement and Variants

Eaglewood is known to Chinese herbalists as *chen xiang* (沉香). Two varieties are sold under this name, *Aquilaria agallocha (a ga ru)* and *Aquilaria sinensis (ar skya)*. The latter has similar properties but is heavier (Pasang Yonten Arya 1998). However, a number of *Aquilaria* species have become threatened because of excessive or incorrect harvesting (IUCN 2009).

Known Pharmacological Properties

Eaglewood has a strong antitubercular action and an antihistaminic action. It also relaxes the smooth muscles (Bensky and Gamble 1986; Chinese Materia Medica 2002).

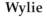

Wylie	*kaNDa ka ri*
Drug name	Two-flowered raspberry
Botanical name	*Rubus biflorus*
Part used	Stalk
Taste and properties	Sweet and acrid; neutral

Traditional Actions and Clinical Uses

- Treats fever associated with wind, disturbed fever, and unripe fever. Two-flowered raspberry is often used in combination with *ma nu pa tra* (elecampane), *sle tres* (moonseed), and *sga skya* (galangal) to treat recently acquired fever, to gather or ripen fever, or to make hidden fever manifest.
- Treats cold disorders, lung disorders, and respiratory disorders.
- Restores vitality.

Procurement and Variants

The leaf of various other plants of the *Rubus* genus, including *R. ellipticus* (yellow Himalayan raspberry) is known as *ga bra* and has very similar actions. Raspberry leaf, common in Western herbalism, is probably a good substitute. Blackberry, a closely related *Rubus* species, may also be considered. Although the name *kaNDa ka ri* is of Indian origin, the Ayurvedic herb *kantkari (Solanum xanthocarpum),* a kind of eggplant, does not have the same action (Tendzin Dakpa 2007).

Known Pharmacological Properties

- Blackberry leaf *(Rubus ulmifolius)* has hypoglycemic, antimicrobial, antiwrinkle, and antioxidant actions.
- Raspberry leaf *(Rubus idaeus)* has antimicrobial, antileukemia, smooth-muscle relaxant, and antioxidant actions.

Additional References

Herrmann, M., S. Grether-Beck, I. Meyer, H. Franke, H. Joppe, J. Krutmann, and G. Vielhaber. 2007. Blackberry leaf extract: A multifunctional antiaging active. *International Journal of Cosmetic Science* 29 (5): 411.

Lemus, I., R. García, E. Delvillar, and G. Knop. 1999. Hypoglycaemic activity of four plants used in Chilean popular medicine. *Phytotherapy Research* 13 (2): 91–4.

Panizzi, L., C. Caponi, S. Catalano, P. L. Cioni, and I. Morelli. 2002. In vitro antimicrobial activity of extracts and isolated constituents of *Rubus ulmifolius. Journal of Ethnopharmacology* 79 (2): 165–8.

Rojas-Vera, J., A. V. Patel, and C. G. Dacke. 2002. Relaxant activity of raspberry (*Rubus idaeus*) leaf extract in guinea-pig ileum in vitro. *Phytotherapy Research* 16 (7): 665–8.

Skupień, K., J. Oszmiański, D. Kostrzewa-Nowak, and J. Tarasiuk. 2006. In vitro antileukaemic activity of extracts from berry plant leaves against sensitive and multidrug resistant HL60 cells. *Cancer Letters* 236 (2): 282–91.

Venskutonis, P. R., A. Dvaranauskaite, and J. Labokas. 2007. Radical scavenging activity and composition of raspberry (*Rubus idaeus*) leaves from different locations in Lithuania. *Fitoterapia* 78 (2): 162–5.

Wang, S. Y., and H. S. Lin. 2000. Antioxidant activity in fruits and leaves of blackberry, raspberry, and strawberry varies with cultivar and developmental stage. *Journal of Agricultural and Food Chemistry* 48 (2): 140–6.

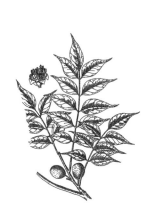

 སྙིང་ཞོ་ཤ་

Wylie	*snying zho sha*
Drug name	Lapsi tree
Botanical name	*Choerospondias axillaris*
Part used	Seeds
Taste and properties	Bitter and sweet; cooling

Traditional Actions and Clinical Uses

Treats heart fever, especially when wind is present.

Known Pharmacological Properties

Lapsi tree has cardiotonic, tachycardic, antiarrhythmic, antithrombotic, and immunostimulant actions. It also helps improve oxygen diffusion in ischemia (Chinese Materia Medica 2002).

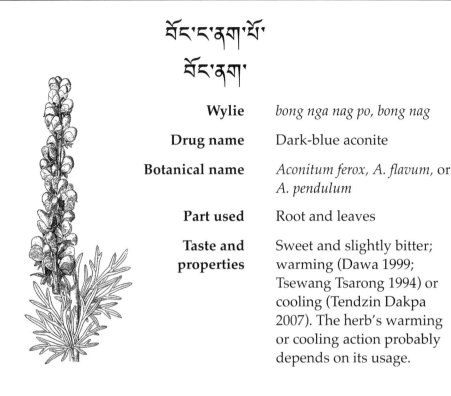

བོང་ང་ནག་པོ་
བོང་ནག་

Wylie	*bong nga nag po, bong nag*
Drug name	Dark-blue aconite
Botanical name	*Aconitum ferox, A. flavum,* or *A. pendulum*
Part used	Root and leaves
Taste and properties	Sweet and slightly bitter; warming (Dawa 1999; Tsewang Tsarong 1994) or cooling (Tendzin Dakpa 2007). The herb's warming or cooling action probably depends on its usage.

Traditional Actions and Clinical Uses

- Relieves joint pain.
- Restores body heat.
- Treats heart wind.

Procurement and Variants

There exist many varieties of aconite, all of which are very toxic. The color designation (*nag po,* meaning "black") refers to the color of the root tissue (Kletter and Kriechbaum 2001). Medicinal aconite may or may not be processed in order to reduce its toxicity. Whether a given type of commercially available aconite is a suitable substitute for *bong nga nag po* must be ascertained very carefully; Kletter and Kriechbaum (2001) discuss the procurement of aconite species. The European variety of dark-blue aconite, *Aconitum napellus,* may be considered.

Known Pharmacological Properties

Dark-blue aconite has an anti-inflammatory action and a very strong analgesic action (Chinese Materia Medica 2002).

གུ་གུལ་

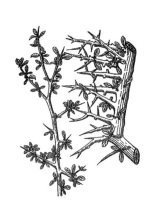

Wylie	*gu gul*
Drug name	Myrrh
Botanical name	*Commiphora mukul*
Part used	Resin
Taste and properties	Bitter and astringent; cooling and heavy

Traditional Actions and Clinical Uses

- Treats disorders caused by *klu* (subterranean or aquatic elemental spirits).
- Treats recent and chronic liver ailments.
- Treats heat and lymph (*chu ser*) disorders.
- Treats infections.

Procurement

Myrrh is available from Ayurvedic herbalists as *guggulu* and from Chinese herbalists as *mo yao* (没药).

Known Pharmacological Properties

Myrrh has hypolipidemic, thyroid stimulant, anti-inflammatory, antithrombotic, cardioprotective, antiarthritic, and antitumor actions (Caldecott 2006; Williamson 2002; WHO 2007).

Additional Reference

Kimura, I., M. Yoshikawa, S. Kobayashi, Y. Sugihara, M. Suzuki, H. Oominami, T. Murakami, H. Matsuda, and V. V. Doiphode. 2001. New triterpenes, myrrhanol A and myrrhanone A, from guggul-gum resins, and their potent anti-inflammatory effect on adjuvant-induced air-pouch granuloma of mice. *Bioorganic and Medicinal Chemistry Letters* 11 (8): 985–9.

 གོ་སྙོད་

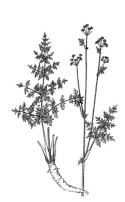

Wylie	*go snyod*
Drug name	Caraway
Botanical name	*Carum carvi*
Part used	Seed
Taste and properties	Sweet, acrid, and astringent; warming and oily

Traditional Actions and Clinical Uses

* Treats fever associated with wind.
* Treats fever in the heart.
* Treats phlegm and restores digestive heat.

Procurement

Caraway is a common spice.

Known Pharmacological Properties

Caraway has antiulcer, antioxidant, hypoglycemic, antibacterial, hypolipidemic, anticancer, and diuretic actions. It also stimulates the production of detoxifying enzymes.

References

Eddouks, M., A. Lemhadri, and J. B. Michel. 2004. Caraway and caper: Potential antihyperglycaemic plants in diabetic rats. *Journal of Ethnopharmacology* 94 (1): 143–8.

Iacobellis, N. S., P. Lo Cantore, F. Capasso, and F. Senatore. 2005. Antibacterial activity of *Cuminum cyminum* L. and *Carum carvi* L. essential oils. *Journal of Agricultural and Food Chemistry* 53 (1): 57–61.

Kamaleeswari, M., K. Deeptha, M. Sengottuvelan, and N. Nalini. 2004. Effect of dietary caraway (*Carum carvi* L.) on aberrant crypt foci development, fecal steroids, and intestinal alkaline phosphatase activities in 1,2-dimethylhydrazine-induced colon carcinogenesis. *Toxicology and Applied Pharmacology* 214 (3): 290–6.

Khayyal, M. T., M. A. el-Ghazaly, S. A. Kenawy, M. Seif-el-Nasr, L. G. Mahran, Y. A. Kafafi, and S. N. Okpanyi. 2001. Antiulcerogenic effect of some gastrointestinally acting plant extracts and their combination. *Arzneimittelforschung* 51 (7): 545–53.

Lahlou, S., A. Tahraoui, Z. Israili, and B. Lyoussi. 2007. Diuretic activity of the aqueous extracts of *Carum carvi* and *Tanacetum vulgare* in normal rats. *Journal of Ethnopharmacology* 110 (3): 458–63.

Lemhadri, A., L. Hajji, J. B. Michel, and M. Eddouks. 2006. Cholesterol and triglycerides lowering activities of caraway fruits in normal and streptozotocin diabetic rats. *Journal of Ethnopharmacology* 106 (3): 321–6.

Satyanarayana, S., K. Sushruta, G. S. Sarma, N. Srinivas, and G. V. Subba Raju. 2004. Antioxidant activity of the aqueous extracts of spicy food additives—evaluation and comparison with ascorbic acid in in-vitro systems. *Journal of Herbal Pharmacotherapy* 4 (2): 1–10.

Zheng, G. Q., P. M. Kenney, and L. K. Lam. 1992. Anethofuran, carvone, and limonene: Potential cancer chemopreventive agents from dill weed oil and caraway oil. *Planta Medica* 58 (4): 338–41.

Herbs That Treat Bile Disorders

ཏིག་ཏ་

Wylie	*tig ta*
Drug name	Chiretta
Botanical name	*Swertia chirayita*
Part used	Aerial part of the plant
Taste and properties	Extremely bitter; cooling, sharp, rough, and blunt

Traditional Actions and Clinical Uses

- Lowers fever associated with bile and blood disorders: this is the most important herb for treating recent or chronic bile disorders, including when other humors are involved. It is also often used in the treatment of dark phlegm, especially if bile or blood is predominant.
- Treats fever of the liver and gallbladder.

Procurement and Variants

Tibetan medicine considers at least three varieties of *tig ta* (Kletter and Kriechbaum 2001; Pasang Yonten Arya 1998). The most common is the Indian variety, *rgya tig* (*Swertia chirayita*), available from Ayurvedic herbalists as *chirayata*. However, it has become threatened in the Indian state of Himachal Pradesh (Badola and Pal 2002).

Known Pharmacological Properties

Indian chiretta (*Swertia chirayita*) has hepatoprotective, anti-inflammatory, anti-ulcer, hypoglycemic, antimicrobial, and antiprotozoal actions (Williamson 2002).

ཀ་ར་

Wylie	*ka ra*
Drug name	White rock sugar
Latin name	*Saccharum purificatum*
Taste and properties	Sweet; cooling and sharp

Traditional Actions and Clinical Uses

- Treats excessive body heat, thirst, nausea, fainting, and bile disorders.
- Serves as a vehicle for preparations used to treat blood and bile disorders.

Procurement

Common refined sugar is adequate.

Remark

Because of the prevalence of cold diseases in modern days, especially diabetes mellitus, sugar is often omitted from formulas that traditionally include it.

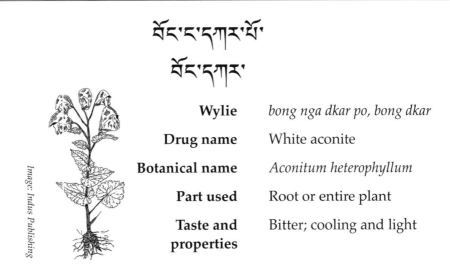

བོང་ང་དཀར་པོ་
བོང་དཀར་

Wylie	*bong nga dkar po, bong dkar*
Drug name	White aconite
Botanical name	*Aconitum heterophyllum*
Part used	Root or entire plant
Taste and properties	Bitter; cooling and light

Image: Indus Publishing

Traditional Actions and Clinical Uses

Treats bile fever and epidemic fever: this is another very important herb in the general treatment of recent or chronic bile and fever disorders.

Procurement and Variants

White aconite is available from Ayurvedic herbalists as *ativisha (Aconitum heterophyllum)*. It has become threatened in the Indian state of Himachal Pradesh (Badola and Pal 2002).

The color designation (*dkar po* means "white") refers to the color of the root tissue (Kletter and Kriechbaum 2001). There exist many varieties of aconite, all of which are very toxic. Medicinal aconite may or may not be processed to reduce its toxicity. Whether a given type of commercially available aconite is a suitable substitute for *bong nga dkar po* must be ascertained very carefully; Kletter and Kriechbaum (2001) discuss the procurement of aconite species.

Known Pharmacological Properties

Aconite's main effect is to raise cell membranes' sodium permeability and to retard repolarization. It has irritant, hypotensive, vasodilatory, anti-inflammatory, depressant, febrifugal, and dose-dependent bradycardic or tachycardic actions. It also has steroid hormone-like effects (Bensky and Gamble 1986).

གསེར་གྱི་མེ་ཏོག་

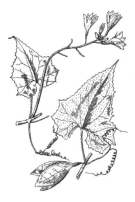

Wylie	*gser gyi me tog*
Drug name	Bolenggua
Botanical name	*Herpetospermum pedunculosum*
Part used	Flower and seed
Taste and properties	Bitter; cooling, sharp, and coarse

Traditional Actions and Clinical Uses

- Treats bile fever: this is one of the most important herbs for the treatment of bile.
- Benefits the spleen, liver, and gallbladder.

Procurement and Variants

Fang et al. suggest that bolenggua *(Herpetospermum pedunculosum)*, bitter melon *(Momordica charantia)* and gac seed *(Momordica cochinchinensis)* have very similar effects. However, gac seed is considered poisonous and is reserved for external use in traditional Chinese medicine (Bensky and Gamble 1986), while the fruit is a common foodstuff in Southeast Asia. Bitter melon is available from Chinese herbalists as *ku gua gan* (苦瓜干) and from Ayurvedic herbalists as *karela.* It can often be purchased fresh in Asian grocery stores. Gac fruit is sometimes available in extract and juice forms from health food stores.

Known Pharmacological Properties

- Bolenggua *(Herpetospermum pedunculosum)* has anti-inflammatory, hepatoprotective, and antioxidant actions.
- Bitter melon is well known for its hypoglycemic properties. It also has abortifacient, antilipolytic, antimicrobial, hepatoprotective, and other actions (Williamson 2002).
- In one study, gac fruit and bitter melon have shown potential anti-HIV action.
- Gac fruit has anticancer, antioxidant, and antiangiogenic actions.

Additional References

Fang, Q. M., H. Zhang, Y. Cao, and C. Wang. 2007. Anti-inflammatory and free radical scavenging activities of ethanol extracts of three seeds used as "Bolengguazi." *Journal of Ethnopharmacology* 114 (1): 61–5.

Momordica charantia (bitter melon) monograph. 2007. *Alternative Medicine Review* 12 (4): 360–3.

Ng, T. B., W. Y. Chan, and H. W. Yeung. 1992. Proteins with abortifacient, ribosome inactivating, immunomodulatory, antitumor, and anti-AIDS activities from *Cucurbitaceae* plants. *General Pharmacology* 23 (4): 579–90.

Tien, P. G., F. Kayama, F. Konishi, H. Tamemoto, K. Kasono, N. T. Hung, M. Kuroki, S. E. Ishikawa, C. N. Van, and M. Kawakami. 2005. Inhibition of tumor growth and angiogenesis by water extract of gac fruit (*Momordica cochinchinensis* Spreng). *International Journal of Oncology* 26 (4): 881–9.

Tsoi, A. Y., T. B. Ng, and W. P. Fong. 2005. Antioxidative effect of a chymotrypsin inhibitor from *Momordica cochinchinensis* (*Cucurbitaceae*) seeds in a primary rat hepatocyte culture. *Journal of Peptide Science* 11 (10): 665–8.

Zhang, M., Y. Deng, H. B. Zhang, X. L. Su, H. L. Chen, T. Yu, and P. Guo. 2008. Two new coumarins from *Herpetospermum caudigerum*. *Chemical and Pharmaceutical Bulletin* 56 (2): 192–3.

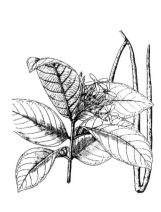

Wylie	*dug mo nyung*
Drug name	Kurchi
Botanical name	*Holarrhena antidysenterica*
Part used	Seed
Taste and properties	Bitter; cooling

Traditional Actions and Clinical Uses

- Treats bile disorders, especially associated with the gallbladder: this is another widely used herb for the treatment of bile disorders.
- Treats dysentery: kurchi is often used in epidemic fever or dark phlegm when the intestines are affected. It is part of the cooling building-block combination called Indra Four (see next chapter).
- Kurchi directs the action of a formula to the small intestine (Dawa 1999).
- Alleviates diarrhea (Thubten Phuntsog 2001).

Procurement

This plant is available from Ayurvedic suppliers as *kurchi*.

Known Pharmacological Properties

Kurchi has marked antibacterial, antiamoebic, antidysentery, and antidiarrheal actions. It has also been found to have immunomodulatory and hypoglycemic actions (Caldecott 2006; Williamson 2002).

བ་ལེ་ཀ་

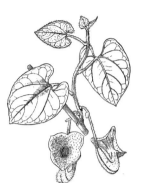

Wylie	*ba le ka*
Drug name	Birthwort
Botanical name	*Aristolochia moupinensis*
Part used	Stem
Taste and properties	Bitter; cooling and coarse

Traditional Actions and Clinical Uses

- Treats hot disorders of the lungs, liver, and intestines.
- Treats blood disorders.

Known Pharmacological Properties

The Ayurvedic variety of birthwort *(Aristolochia indica)* has antifertility, antiestrogenic, abortifacient, antitumor, immunomodulatory, and anti-inflammatory actions (Williamson 2002).

Remark

There is some controversy concerning the use of various plants of the genus *Aristolochia* because of the nephrotoxicity and carcinogenicity of the aristolochic acids.

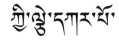

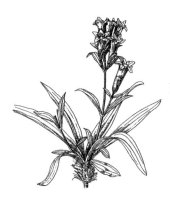

Wylie	*kyi lce dkar po*
Drug name	Broad-leaf gentian
Botanical name	*Gentiana robusta* or *G. straminea*
Part used	Flower
Taste and properties	Bitter; cooling

Traditional Actions and Clinical Uses

- Treats bile disorders and hot disorders of the stomach, liver, and gallbladder: broad-leaf gentian is often used in combination with *tig ta* (chiretta), *gser gyi me tog* (bolenggua), and/or *dug mo nyung* (kurchi).
- Heals wounds and reduces swelling.

Procurement and Variants

There exist several varieties of broad-leaf gentian, collectively known to Chinese botanists as *qin jiao* (秦艽), the root of which is available from Chinese herbalists. Its clinical effects are probably similar to those of the aerial part of the plant.

Known Pharmacological Properties

The root of the Chinese variety of broad-leaf gentian has anti-inflammatory, sedative, analgesic, antipyretic, antianaphylactic, antihistaminic, hyperglycemic, hypotensive, bradycardic, and bacteriostatic actions (Chang and But 1987).

རྩ་མཁྲིས་

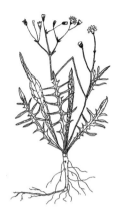

Wylie	*rtsa mkhris*
Drug name	Rabbit milkweed
Botanical name	*Ixeris chinensis* or *I. gracilis; Saussurea graminea* or *S. eopygmaea*
Part used	Aerial part of the plant
Taste and properties	Bitter; cooling

Traditional Actions and Clinical Uses

- Treats bile disorders.
- Treats wind diseases, especially cold.
- Treats heart disorders.
- Helps digestion.

Known Pharmacological Properties

Rabbit milkweed reduces the heart rate and heart contraction in rabbits but increases heart contraction in frogs. It has vasodilatory, adrenergic, and hypotensive actions mediated by the central nervous system (Chinese Materia Medica 2002).

Remark

Rabbit milkweed has cold postdigestive power and therefore can harm the kidneys.

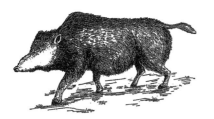

Wylie	*gar nag*
Drug name	Calcined wild-boar stool
Latin name	*Excrementum sus scrofae*
Taste and properties	Salty; cooling

Traditional Actions and Clinical Uses

- Treats indigestion.
- Treats bile tumors.
- Treats epidemic fever.

Procurement and Variants

The stool of organically raised farm pigs is probably a good substitute for wild-boar stool.

Known Pharmacological Properties

Wild boar bile has anti-inflammatory, analgesic, and cholesterol-reducing actions. It improves the absorption of calcium, penicillin, and aspirin (Chinese Materia Medica 2002).

ཌོང་ག་

Wylie	*dong ga*
Drug name	Golden shower tree
Botanical name	*Cassia fistula*
Part used	Seeds and pods
Taste and properties	Sweet and acrid; cooling, heavy, and oily

Traditional Actions and Clinical Uses

- Treats bile disorders associated with the stomach and liver.
- Detoxifies.
- Reduces swelling in the limbs.

Procurement

Golden shower tree may be available from Ayurvedic sources as *aragvadha*.

Known Pharmacological Properties

Golden shower tree has laxative, intestinal stimulant, antibacterial, antiviral, and antifungal actions. In one study, it improved prolapsed heart valves in rabbits (Chinese Materia Medica 2002).

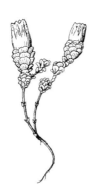

གང་གུ་ཆུང་

Wylie	*gang gA chung*
Botanical name	*Gentiana urnula*
Part used	Flower
Taste and properties	Bitter; cooling

Traditional Actions and Clinical Uses

- Treats poisoning, infectious common cold, and dysentery.
- Treats hot blood disorders.
- Benefits the gallbladder.
- Treats complex disorders that involve wind, bile, phlegm, blood, and lymph (*chu ser*).

Herbs That Treat Blood and Lymph Disorders

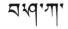

Wylie	*ba sha ka*
Drug name	Malabar nut tree
Botanical name	*Justicia adhatoda* syn. *Adhatoda vasica*
Part used	Twig, leaf, flower, and seed
Taste and properties	Bitter; cooling, light, and blunt

Traditional Actions and Clinical Uses

- Treats fever of the blood, bile, and liver: this herb has a broad range of uses in the treatment of bile, blood, fever, and dark-phlegm conditions. It is also used in decoctions that gather fever.
- Malabar nut tree directs the action of a formula to the blood (Dawa 1999).

Procurement

Malabar nut tree is available from Ayurvedic herbalists as *vasaka*.

Known Pharmacological Properties

Malabar nut tree has bronchodilatory, antiasthmatic, antibacterial, anti-inflammatory, antiallergenic, antitubercular, cholagogic, digestant, abortifacient, uterotonic, and vulnerary actions (Caldecott 2006; Williamson 2002).

ཀོང་ལེན་

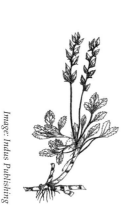

Image: Indus Publishing

Wylie	*hong len*
Drug name	Picrorhiza grass
Botanical name	*Picrorhiza sp.* or *Lagotis sp.*
Part used	Root or entire plant
Taste and properties	Bitter and astringent; cooling and coarse

Traditional Actions and Clinical Uses

- Treats blood and bile disorders and fever in the vital organs: this herb has very broad uses in the treatment of bile, blood, and fever disorders.
- Detoxifies.

Procurement and Variants

Picrorhiza grass is available from Ayurvedic herbalists as *kutaki* and from Chinese herbalists as *hu huang lian* (胡黄连). There exist many variants of this herb, especially within the *Lagotis* genus (Kletter and Kriechbaum 2001). *Picrorhiza kurroa* has become threatened in the Indian state of Himachal Pradesh (Badola and Pal 2002).

Known Pharmacological Properties

Picrorhiza grass has hepatoprotective, choleretic, immunomodulatory, anti-inflammatory, antioxidant, antiasthmatic, cardioprotective, hypoglycemic, and other actions (Caldecott 2006; Williamson 2002).

Additional Reference

Picrorhiza kurroa monograph. 2001. *Alternative Medicine Review* 6 (3): 319–21.

ཙན་དན་དམར་པོ་

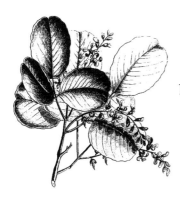

Wylie	*tsan dan dmar po*
Drug name	Red sandalwood
Botanical name	*Pterocarpus santalinus*
Part used	Wood
Taste and properties	Astringent, slightly bitter; cooling

Traditional Actions and Clinical Uses

- Treats blood fever.
- Treats combined blood and wind disorders.

Procurement

Red sandalwood is known to Ayurvedic herbalists as *rakta chandana,* but it is threatened (IUCN 2009) as a result of excessive harvesting.

Known Pharmacological Properties

In one study, red sandalwood relieved cancer-related ascites (Chinese Materia Medica 2002). Hypoglycemic action has been noted (Gruenwald et al. 2000).

རྒྱ་སྐྱེགས་
རྒྱ་ཚོས་
ཚོས་

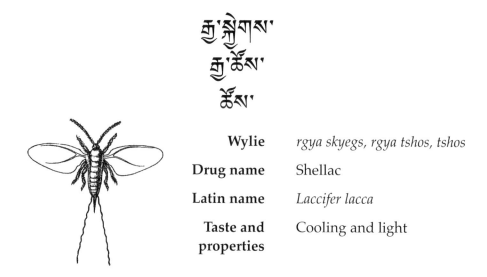

Wylie	*rgya skyegs, rgya tshos, tshos*
Drug name	Shellac
Latin name	*Laccifer lacca*
Taste and properties	Cooling and light

Traditional Actions and Clinical Uses

Treats blood and fever disorders: shellac is often used for cooling the blood, in the treatment of dark-phlegm conditions, or to remove heat from the lungs or from the kidneys.

Procurement

Shellac is the secretion of one of possibly several insects that live on the sap of selected trees. It is a nontoxic natural wood finishing product available from wood-finish vendors. The garnet-colored wax-free flakes are probably the most suitable form. Liquid shellac, based on denatured alcohol, is not suitable for human consumption.

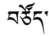

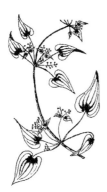

Wylie	*btsod*
Drug name	Indian madder
Botanical name	*Rubia cordifolia*
Part used	Roots and stems
Taste and properties	Acrid and bitter; cooling

Traditional Actions and Clinical Uses

- Treats blood disorders.
- Treats spread fever.
- Treats fever of the lungs, kidneys, and intestines.
- Reduces swelling.
- Indian madder is used in combination with *rgya skyegs* (shellac), *'bri mog* (Tibetan groomwell), and / or *zhu mkhan* (sapphireberry) to treat fever in the blood and in the lungs and to remove heat from the kidneys.

Procurement

Indian madder is available from Ayurvedic herbalists as *manjista* and from Chinese herbalists as *qian cao gen* (茜草根).

Known Pharmacological Properties

Indian madder has antioxidant, anti-inflammatory, antiplatelet, hemostatic, antibacterial, vasodilatory, anticancer, antitussive, expectorant, hepatoprotective, and other effects (Bensky and Gamble 1986; Caldecott 2006; Chang and But 1987; Williamson 2002).

རེ་སྐོན་

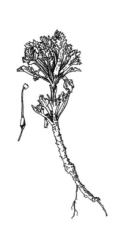

Wylie	*re skon*
Drug name	Nepalese fumewort
Botanical name	*Corydalis hendersonii* or *C. nepalensis*
Part used	Entire plant
Taste and properties	Extremely bitter; cooling

Traditional Actions and Clinical Uses

- Treats blood disorders.
- Treats fever in the channels caused by dark phlegm.

Procurement and Variants

Nepalese fumewort is hard to obtain. The suitability of other members of the *Corydalis* genus must be researched.

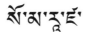

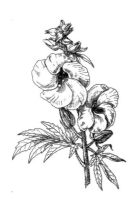

Wylie	*so ma rA dza*
Drug name	Aibika
Botanical name	*Abelmoschus manihot*
Part used	Seed
Taste and properties	Astringent, bitter, and slightly acrid; warming

Traditional Actions and Clinical Uses

- Treats leukorrhea.
- Treats skin disorders.
- Acts as an aphrodisiac.
- Controls sweating.
- Treats diabetes.
- Aibika is used in the treatment of turbid fever and blood disorders.
- Treats lymph *(chu ser)* disorders when used in combination with *spos dkar* (frankincense) and *thal ka rdo rje* (foetid cassia).

Procurement and Variants

Aibika seed is sometimes available from seed vendors. A closely related species, *Abelmoschus moschatus,* may be available from Ayurvedic herbalists as *latakasturi.*

Known Pharmacological Properties

Aibika has neuroprotective, antiviral, nephroprotective, and antithrombotic actions. It can also prevent bone loss.

Remark

The Tibetan herb name *so ma rA dza* is sometimes associated with the seed of marijuana *(Cannabis sativa),* but the latter has a different action and is more correctly called *sro ma ra tsa, sro ma ra tsa nag po,* or *sro ma nag po* (Pasang Yonten Arya 1998; Tendzin Dakpa 2007).

Additional References

Cheng, X. P., S. Qin, L. Y. Dong, and J. N. Zhou. 2006. Inhibitory effect of total flavone of *Abelmoschus manihot* L. Medic on NMDA receptor–mediated current in cultured rat hippocampal neurons. *Neuroscience Research* 55 (2): 142–5.

Guo, Y., L. Fan, L. Y. Dong, and Z. W. Chen. 2005. Effects of total flavone of *Abelmoschl manihot* L. Medic on the function of platelets and its mechanism. *Chinese Journal of Integrative Medicine* 11 (1): 57–9.

Puel, C., J. Mathey, S. Kati-Coulibaly, M. J. Davicco, P. Lebecque, B. Chanteranne, M. N. Horcajada, and V. Coxam. 2005. Preventive effect of *Abelmoschus manihot* (L.) Medik. on bone loss in the ovariectomised rats. *Journal of Ethnopharmacology* 99 (1): 55–60.

Wen, J. Y., and Z. W. Chen. 2007. Protective effect of pharmacological preconditioning of total flavones of *Abelmoschl manihot* on cerebral ischemic reperfusion injury in rats. *American Journal of Chinese Medicine* 35 (4): 653–61.

Wu, L. L., X. B. Yang, Z. M. Huang, H. Z. Liu, and G. X. Wu. 2007. In vivo and in vitro antiviral activity of hyperoside extracted from *Abelmoschus manihot* (L) Medik. *Acta Pharmacologica Sinica* 28 (3): 404–9.

Yu, J. Y., and N. N. Xiong. 1992. Pathogenic factor (dampness-heat) of glomerulopathy (in Chinese). *Zhongguo Zhong Xi Yi Jie He Za Zhi* 12 (8): 458–60, 451.

Yu, J. Y., and N. N. Xiong. 1993. Relation between dampness-heat syndrome of glomerulonephritis and sialic acid and N-acetyl-beta-D-glucosaminidase (NAG). *Zhongguo Zhong Xi Yi Jie He Za Zhi* 13 (9): 525–7, 515–6.

Yu, J. Y., N. N. Xiong, and H. F. Guo. 1995. Clinical observation on diabetic nephropathy treated with alcohol of *Abelmoschus manihot* (in Chinese). *Zhongguo Zhong Xi Yi Jie He Za Zhi* 15 (5): 263–5.

ཐལ་ཀ་རྡོ་རྗེ་

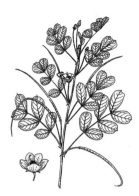

Wylie	*thal ka rdo rje*
Drug name	Foetid cassia
Botanical name	*Cassia tora*
Part used	Seed
Taste and properties	Bitter and astringent; cool and coarse

Traditional Actions and Clinical Uses

- Treats skin disorders.
- Treats lymph *(chu ser)* disorders, often in combination with *so ma rA dza* (aibika) and *spos dkar* (frankincense).
- Acts as an aphrodisiac.

Procurement

Foetid cassia is available from Chinese herbalists as *jue ming zi* (决明子).

Known Pharmacological Properties

Foetid cassia has antibacterial, hypotensive, analgesic, antiatherosclerotic, anti-thrombotic, immunostimulant, hepatoprotective, detoxifying, and antidiarrheal actions. It can lower triglycerides and increase HDL cholesterol. One of its constituents was noted as potentially carcinogenic (Chinese Materia Medica 2002).

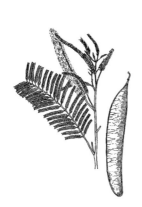

སེང་ལྡེང་

Wylie	*seng ldeng*
Drug name	Catechu tree
Botanical name	*Acacia catechu*
Part used	Concentrated extract
Taste and properties	Astringent and bitter; cooling

Traditional Actions and Clinical Uses

Treats blood and lymph *(chu ser)* disorders. Catechu tree is used in the treatment of chronic fever and turbid fever.

Procurement

Catechu tree is available from Ayurvedic herbalists as *khadira*. Chinese medicine uses catechu tree interchangeably with gambir *(Uncaria gambir)*. The extract of either tree is available from Chinese herbalists under the drug name *er cha* (儿茶).

Known Pharmacological Properties

Catechu tree has hepatoprotective, anti-inflammatory, antifungal, and hypocalcemic actions. It may also have a beneficial effect on leukemia (Williamson 2002).

ཁྲེ་ག་

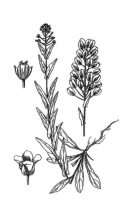

Wylie	*bre ga*
Drug name	Pennycress
Botanical name	*Thlaspi arvense*
Part used	Seed or leaf and stem
Taste and properties	Bitter and acrid; warming, oily, and dry

Traditional Actions and Clinical Uses

- Treats lung and kidney disorders.
- Treats leukorrhea.
- Helps restore the appetite.
- Relieves accumulation of serous fluid in the joints.

Procurement

Pennycress seeds may be available from seed vendors.

Known Pharmacological Properties

Pennycress helps reduce uric acid and is thus useful in the treatment of gout. It also has an antibacterial action (Chinese Materia Medica 2002).

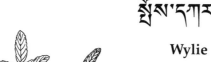

 སྤོས་དཀར་

Wylie	*spos dkar*
Drug name	Frankincense
Botanical name	*Boswellia carterii* or *B. serrata*
Part used	Resin
Taste and properties	Warming and dry

Traditional Actions and Clinical Uses

- Treats lymph *(chu ser)* disorders, often in combination with *so ma rA dza* (aibika) and *thal ka rdo rje* (foetid cassia).
- Frankincense, through its action on the lymph *(chu ser)*, benefits the heart indirectly and is used in formulas that treat heart wind.

Procurement

Medicinal frankincense is available from Chinese herbalists as *ru xiang* (乳香) and from Ayurvedic herbalists as *sallaki*.

Known Pharmacological Properties

Frankincense has anti-inflammatory, antiarthritic, analgesic, hypolipidemic, im-munomodulatory, antitumor, antiasthmatic, and antifungal actions (Williamson 2002).

Additional Reference

Boswellia serrata monograph. 2008. *Alternative Medicine Review* 13 (2): 165–8.

ཚ་ལ་

Wylie	*tsha la*
Drug name	Borax
Taste and properties	Sweet and salty; neutral

Traditional Actions and Clinical Uses

- Heals wounds.
- Dissolves blood clots.
- Works as a purgative.
- Dries up lymph *(chu ser)*.

Chemical Composition

Sodium borate, $Na_2B_4O_7$

Procurement

Medicinal borax is available from Chinese herbalists as *peng sha* (硼砂).

Known Pharmacological Properties

Borax has antibacterial and anticonvulsive actions (Chinese Materia Medica 2002).

Herbs That Treat Fever

Wylie	*gi waM, gi wang*
Drug name	Elephant or ox gallstone
Latin name	*Barrus sp.* or *Bovus sp.*
Part used	Gallstone
Taste and properties	Bitter; cooling

Traditional Actions and Clinical Uses

- Treats epidemic illnesses and poisoning.
- Treats liver disorders.
- Treats fever of the channels.
- Elephant or ox gallstone is especially suited for mild fevers: compare with *ga bur* (camphor) and *tsan dan dkar po* (white sandalwood). It may be taken with water for all kinds of fever (Thubten Phuntsog 2001).

Procurement

Ox gallstone is available from Chinese herbalists as *niu huang* (牛黄).

Known Pharmacological Properties

Ox gallstone has anticonvulsant, antimicrobial, anti-inflammatory, antiallergic, antidotal, hypotensive, erythropoietic, anticancer, and choleretic actions (Chang and But 1986).

ཙན་དན་དཀར་པོ་

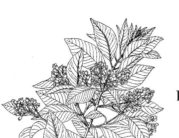

Wylie	*tsan dan dkar po*
Drug name	White sandalwood
Botanical name	*Santalum album*
Part used	Wood
Taste and properties	Astringent; cooling

Traditional Actions and Clinical Uses

- Treats fever of the heart and lungs.
- Treats disturbed fever.
- Sandalwood is especially suited for moderate fevers: compare with *gi waM* (elephant or ox gallstone) and *ga bur* (camphor).

Procurement

Sandalwood is known to Ayurvedic herbalists as *chandana* and to Chinese herbalists as *tan xiang* (檀香). However, it has recently become threatened by excessive harvesting (IUCN 2009).

Known Pharmacological Properties

Sandalwood has hepatoprotective, antitumor, hypotensive, antibacterial, anti-HSV-1, and anti-HSV-2 actions (Caldecott 2006).

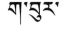

ག་བུར་

Wylie	*ga bur*
Drug name	Camphor
Botanical name	*Cinnamomum camphora*
Part used	Resin
Taste and properties	Acrid, bitter, and astringent; cooling and coarse

Traditional Actions and Clinical Uses

- Instantly reduces high fever and chronic fever that has penetrated the bones. Camphor is especially suited for strong fevers: compare with *gi waM* (elephant or ox gallstone) and *tsan dan dkar po* (white sandalwood).
- Relieves severe pain caused by fever.

Procurement

Camphor is available in pharmacies and from Chinese herbalists as *zhang nao* (樟腦).

Known Pharmacological Properties

Camphor has local irritant and antiseptic actions. Taken internally, it is a CNS stimulant, a cardiotonic, a vasoconstrictor of core blood vessels, but a vasodilator of peripheral vessels (Bensky and Gamble 1986). It also has sedative, analgesic, anti-inflammatory, antibacterial, and uterotonic actions. It stimulates contractions of the duodenum and helps the proliferation of nerve cells (Chinese Materia Medica 2002).

Remark

Camphor is toxic in doses as low as 0.5 g.

Wylie	*ut pal*
Drug name	Himalayan poppy
Botanical name	*Meconopsis integrifolia, M. punicea,* or *M. torquata*
Part used	Flower, seed, and leaf
Taste and properties	Sweet and astringent; cooling

Traditional Actions and Clinical Uses

Treats many fever and infectious disorders. Himalayan poppy is often used as an adjunct in the treatment of chronic fever, bile affecting the muscles, dark phlegm, and hot liver disorders.

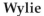

Wylie	*nA ga ge sar*
Drug name	Silk cotton tree
Botanical name	*Bombax ceiba* syn. *B. malabaricum, Gossampinus malabarica*
Part used	Flower
Taste and properties	Astringent; cooling and coarse

Traditional Actions and Clinical Uses

Treats hot disorders of the lungs, heart, and liver.

Procurement and Variants

Silk cotton tree flower is available from Chinese herbalists as *mu mian hua* (木棉花). It should not be confused with ironwood tree, known in Ayurveda as *nagkeshar* (Chinese Materia Medica 2002; Dawa 1999; Pasang Yonten Arya 1998; Tendzin Dakpa 2007).

Known Pharmacological Properties

Silk cotton tree has cardiotonic, antibacterial, and hepatoprotective actions (Chinese Materia Medica 2002).

Remark

Of the "three *ge sar*" (three different parts of the silk cotton tree flower) *nA ga ge sar* is the more common. The "three *ge sar*" also include *pad ma ge sar* and *puShpa ge sar.* They are often used in combination.

མཚལ་

Wylie	*mtshal*
Drug name	Cinnabar
Latin name	*Cinnabaris*
Taste and properties	Slightly sweet, astringent; cooling

Traditional Actions and Clinical Uses

- Heals wounds: applied locally, cinnabar is considered the best remedy to heal suppurating sores and wounds (Thubten Phuntsog 2001).
- Treats fever of the lungs, liver, and channels.

Chemical Composition

Red mercuric sulfide, HgS

Procurement

Cinnabar is available from Chinese herbalists as *zhu sha* (朱砂).

Known Pharmacological Properties

Applied externally, cinnabar has bactericidal and antiparasitic actions. Taken internally, it increases the output of urinary nitrogen (Chinese Materia Medica 2002). It also has a sedative action and has shown an antifertility action on female rats.

Remark

Elemental mercury and organic mercury are highly toxic, but mercury salts, when processed and administered appropriately, are not. Describing the detoxification of mercury and its salts is beyond the scope of this work.

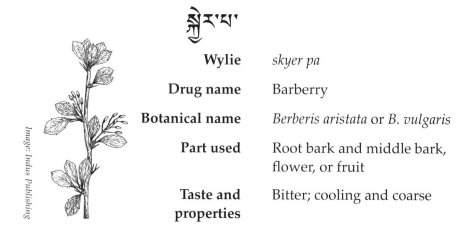

�སྐྱེར་པ་

Wylie	*skyer pa*
Drug name	Barberry
Botanical name	*Berberis aristata* or *B. vulgaris*
Part used	Root bark and middle bark, flower, or fruit
Taste and properties	Bitter; cooling and coarse

Image: Indus Publishing

Traditional Actions and Clinical Uses

- Benefits the eyes: barberry is very effective for a wide range of eye disorders. It can be used in combination with *a ru ra* (chebulic myrobalan) for problems due to toxins, *ba ru ra* (beleric myrobalan) for bile disorders, or *skyu ru ra* (amla) for blood disorders (Thubten Phuntsog 2001).
- Gathers toxins.
- Treats lymph *(chu ser)* disorders.
- Treats chronic fever.
- Helps heal sores.

Procurement and Variants

Barberry can be obtained from Ayurvedic herbalists as *daru haridra*. Barberry berries can be found in Middle Eastern grocery stores. Barberry root bark is available from Western herbalists. The middle bark is the preferred part in Tibetan medicine. It is called *skyer pa'i bar shun*.

Known Pharmacological Properties

Barberry as antibiotic, hepatoprotective, antidiarrheal, anti-inflammatory, and antiplatelet actions (Williamson 2002).

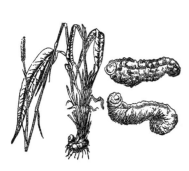

ब्ल'स्नर'

Wylie	*gla sgang*
Drug name	Bistort
Botanical name	*Polygonum bistorta*
Part used	Root
Taste and properties	Acrid, astringent; cooling

Traditional Actions and Clinical Uses

- Treats hot dysentery and epidemic fever: along with *par pa ta* (fumitory), this is an important herb for the treatment of epidemic fever.
- Treats phlegm.
- Treats the lungs and intestines.

Procurement

Bistort is sometimes available from Chinese herbalists as *quan shen* (拳参) or as *cao he che* (草河车).

Known Pharmacological Properties

Bistort has anti-inflammatory and interferon-inducing actions.

References

Duwiejua, M., I. J. Zeitlin, A. I. Gray, and P. G. Waterman. 1999. The anti-inflammatory compounds of *Polygonum bistorta*: Isolation and characterisation. *Planta Medica* 65 (4): 371–4.

Duwiejua, M., I. J. Zeitlin, P. G. Waterman, and A. I. Gray. 1994. Anti-inflammatory activity of *Polygonum bistorta, Guaiacum officinale* and *Hamamelis virginiana* in rats. *Journal of Pharmacy and Pharmacology* 46 (4): 286–90.

Smolarz, H. D., and T. Skwarek. 1999. The investigations into the interferon-like activity of *Polygonum* L. genus. *Acta Poloniae Pharmaceutica* 56 (6): 459–62.

ཡུང་བ་

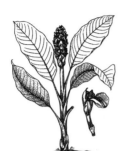

Wylie	*yung ba*
Drug name	Turmeric
Botanical name	*Curcuma longa*
Part used	Root
Taste and properties	Slightly bitter; warming

Traditional Actions and Clinical Uses

- Treats infectious disorders.
- Removes toxins.
- Stops tissue necrosis.

Procurement

Turmeric is a common spice.

Known Pharmacological Properties

Turmeric has numerous beneficial effects, including antiallergic, anti-inflammatory, antibiotic, antioxidant, antispasmodic, antiulcer, antiviral, hepatoprotective, hypoglycemic, antitumor, immunostimulant, antiasthmatic, hypolipidemic, neuroprotective, antimicrobial, antithrombotic, etc. actions (Caldecott 2006; Ross 1999; Williamson 2002).

Additional Reference

Curcuma longa (turmeric) monograph. 2001. *Alternative Medicine Review* 6 (supplement): S62–6.

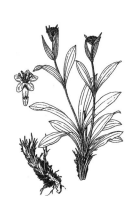

སྤང་སྤོས་

Wylie	*spang spos*
Drug name	Muskroot
Botanical name	*Nardostachys jatamansi*
Part used	Entire plant
Taste and properties	Bitter; cooling

Traditional Actions and Clinical Uses

- Treats poisoning and chronic fever.
- Treats spleen disorders.
- Reduces swelling.

Procurement and Variants

Muskroot is available from Ayurvedic herbalists as *jatamansi*. A related species, *Nardostachys chinensis*, is available from Chinese herbalists as *gan song* (甘松). It has become threatened in the Indian state of Himachal Pradesh (Badola and Pal 2002).

Known Pharmacological Properties

Muskroot has serotonergic, dopaminergic, hypnotic, anticonvulsant, neuroprotective, hepatoprotective, and antioxidant actions (Caldecott 2006).

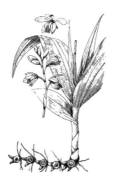

Wylie	*pa to la*
Drug name	Hyacinth orchid
Botanical name	*Bletilla striata*
Part used	Root
Taste and properties	Sweet, bitter, and acrid; sharp

Traditional Actions and Clinical Uses

- Improves the appetite.
- Treats diseases caused by parasites.
- Hyacinth orchid is mentioned in the Oral Instruction Tantra in the treatment of epidemic fever.

Procurement and Variants

Hyacinth orchid is available from Chinese herbalists as *bai ji* (白及).

Known Pharmacological Properties

Hyacinth orchid has hemostatic, antiulcer, antitubercular, and antitussive actions (Bensky and Gamble 1986).

འབུ་སུ་ཧང་

Wylie	*'bu su hang*
Drug name	Alfalfa
Botanical name	*Medicago sativa*
Part used	Aerial part of the plant
Taste and properties	Bitter; cooling

Traditional Actions and Clinical Uses

- Treats hot lung disorders and cough.
- Heals wounds.

Procurement and Variants

Alfalfa leaf is available from Western herbalists.

Known Pharmacological Properties

Alfalfa seed has hypolipidemic, estrogenic, antiatherosclerotic, and hypoglycemic actions. It is not clear whether the seeds have the same effects as the aerial part of the plat.

Remark

Alfalfa seeds and sprouts may produce adverse reactions in patients with SLE or other autoimmune disorders and even trigger SLE-like reactions in healthy patients. Such reactions have been prevented by autoclaving the seeds.

References

Boué, S. M., T. E. Wiese, S. Nehls, M. E. Burow, S. Elliott, C. H. Carter-Wientjes, B. Y. Shih, J. A. McLachlan, and T. E. Cleveland. 2003. Evaluation of the estrogenic effects of legume extracts containing phytoestrogens. *Journal of Agricultural and Food Chemistry* 51 (8): 2193–9.

Malinow, M. R., E. J. Bardana Jr., B. Pirofsky, S. Craig, and P. McLaughlin. 1982. Systemic lupus erythematosus–like syndrome in monkeys fed alfalfa sprouts: Role of a nonprotein amino acid. *Science* 216 (4544): 415–7.

Malinow, M. R., P. McLaughlin, E. J. Bardana Jr., and S. Craig. 1984. Elimination of toxicity from diets containing alfalfa seeds. *Food and Chemical Toxicology* 22 (7): 583–7.

Malinow, M. R., P. McLaughlin, H. K. Naito, L. A. Lewis, and W. P. McNulty. (1978) Effect of alfalfa meal on shrinkage (regression) of atherosclerotic plaques during cholesterol feeding in monkeys. *Atherosclerosis* 30 (1): 27–43.

Mölgaard, J., H. von Schenck, and A. G. Olsson. (1987) Alfalfa seeds lower low density lipoprotein cholesterol and apolipoprotein B concentrations in patients with type II hyperlipoproteinemia. *Atherosclerosis* 65 (1–2): 173–9.

Srinivasan, S. R., D. Patton, B. Radhakrishnamurthy, T. A. Foster, M. R. Malinow, P. McLaughlin, and G. S. Berenson. 1980. Lipid changes in atherosclerotic aortas of *Macaca fascicularis* after various regression regimens. *Atherosclerosis* 37 (4): 591–601.

Swanston-Flatt, S. K., C. Day, C. J. Bailey, and P. R. Flatt. (1990) Traditional plant treatments for diabetes. Studies in normal and streptozotocin diabetic mice. *Diabetologia* 33 (8): 462–4.

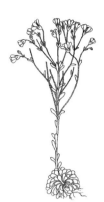

 སུམ་ཅུ་ཏིག་

Wylie	*sum cu tig*
Drug name	Lhasa saxifrage
Botanical name	*Saxifraga lhasana* or *S. umbellulata*
Part used	Entire plant
Taste and properties	Bitter; cooling

Traditional Actions and Clinical Uses

Treats bile disorders and hot disorders of the blood, liver, and gallbladder.

Variant

Tibetan medicine considers *sum cu tig* to be similar to *tig ta* (chiretta) (Pasang Yonten Arya 1998). Some variants of *tig ta* belong to other members of the *Saxifraga* genus (Kletter and Kriechbaum 2001; Pasang Yonten Arya 1998).

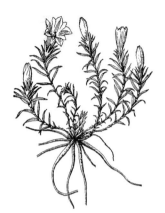

Wylie	*spang rgyan*
Drug name	Small-leaf gentian
Botanical name	*Gentiana algida, G. sino-ornata,* or *G. veichtiorum*
Part used	Flower or entire aerial part of the plant
Taste and properties	Bitter and slightly astringent; cooling

Traditional Actions and Clinical Uses

- Treats infectious and toxic fever.
- Treats infections of the throat and lungs.

Procurement and Variants

There exist several varieties of small-leaf gentian, collectively known to Chinese botanists as *long dan* (龙胆). The root is available from Chinese herbalists as *long dan cao* (龙胆草). Its clinical effects are probably similar to those of the aerial part of the plant.

Known Pharmacological Properties

The root of Chinese small-leaf gentian has stomachic, hepatoprotective, choleretic, diuretic, hypotensive, sedative, analgesic, antidotal, anti-inflammatory, antibacterial, and antiprotozoal actions (Chang and But 1986).

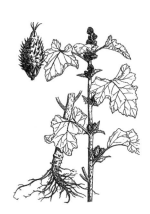

ঠ্র'ৰ্ঠ্রুম

Wylie	*byi tsher*
Drug name	Cocklebur
Botanical name	*Xanthium strumarium* or *X. sibiricum*
Part used	Aerial part of the plant
Taste and properties	Bitter; cooling, slightly poisonous

Traditional Actions and Clinical Uses

- Treats the common cold, toxic fever, and epidemic fever.
- Treats fever of the kidneys.

Procurement

Cocklebur is available from Chinese herbalists as *cang er cao* (苍耳草).

Known Pharmacological Properties

Cocklebur has an anticancer action and a significant antibacterial action (Chang and But 1986). It also has cardiotonic and hypotensive actions and lowers the excitability threshold of the central nervous system (Chinese Materia Medica 2002).

སྤ་སེང་

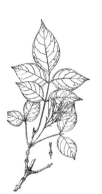

Wylie	*stab seng*
Drug name	Korean ash
Botanical name	*Fraxinus rhynchophylla*
Part used	Branch bark
Taste and properties	Astringent and bitter; cooling

Traditional Actions and Clinical Uses

- Heals broken bones.
- Alleviates stomach pain.

Procurement

Korean ash bark is available from Chinese herbalists as *qin pi* (秦皮).

Known Pharmacological Properties

Korean ash has antibacterial, anti-inflammatory, antitussive, expectorant, anti-asthmatic, sedative, anticonvulsant, and analgesic actions (Chang and But 1987).

ཨ་བྱག་གཟེར་འཇོམས་

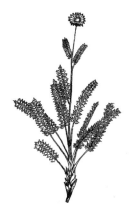

Wylie	*a byag gzer 'joms*
Drug name	Tartar chrysanthemum
Botanical name	*Chrysanthemum tatsienense* syn. *Pyrethrum tatsienense*, *Tanacetum tatsienense*
Part used	Flower
Taste and properties	Bitter; cooling

Traditional Actions and Clinical Uses

- Removes pain in the ribs and upper back.
- Heals broken bones and wounds.
- Reduces excess serous fluids.

Procurement and Variants

Almost nothing is known about the identification of this herb within modern botany. No evidence could be found of either similarity or dissimilarity with other varieties of chrysanthemum in terms of pharmacological action.

Known Pharmacological Properties

Tartar chrysanthemum has antibacterial action (Chinese Materia Medica 2002).

 མཚེ་ལྡུམ་

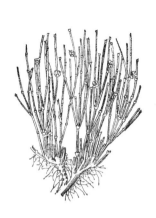

Wylie	*mtshe ldum*
Drug name	Ephedra or ma huang
Botanical name	*Ephedra sp.*
Part used	Leaf, stem, flower, and seed
Taste and properties	Bitter, acrid, and astringent; cooling, light, and coarse

Traditional Actions and Clinical Uses

- Treats recent and chronic fever disorders.
- Rejuvenates.
- Treats hemorrhage.
- Treats hot gallbladder, liver, and spleen disorders.

Procurement

Ephedra is available from Chinese herbalists as *ma huang* (麻黃) and from Western herbalists as either ma huang or ephedra.

Known Pharmacological Properties

Ephedra has numerous sympathomimetic effects and is a very strong CNS stimulant, a febrifuge, an antimicrobial, and an antitussive (Chang and But 1987).

Remark

Ephedra is contraindicated in hypertensive patients.

ཚེར་སྔོན་

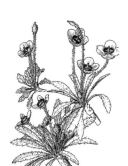

Wylie	*tsher sngon*
Drug name	Blue poppy
Botanical name	*Meconopsis sp.*
Part used	Entire plant
Taste and properties	Bitter; cooling, sharp

Traditional Actions and Clinical Uses

- Strengthens the bones and heals fractured bones, especially those of the skull.
- Lowers bone fever.
- Relieves pain in the chest and upper back.

Procurement and Variants

The flower of the corn poppy *(Papaver rhoeas)* is known as *rgya men me tog* in Tibetan medicine and has comparable actions (Tendzin Dakpa 2007).

Known Pharmacological Properties

Corn poppy has sedative properties and may be of value in the treatment of opiate addiction. Opium poppy has well-known analgesic, hypnotic, respiratory depressant, vasodilatory, and antidiarrheal actions (Bensky and Gamble 1986), although this is not necessarily relevant to the application of blue poppy in Tibetan medicine.

Additional References

El-Masry, S., M. G. El-Ghazooly, A. A. Omar, S. M. Khafagy, and J. D. Phillipson. 1981. Alkaloids from Egyptian *Papaver rhoeas*. *Planta Medica* 41 (1): 61–4.

Pourmotabbed, A., B. Rostamian, G. Manouchehri, G. Pirzadeh-Jahromi, H. Sahraei, H. Ghoshooni, H. Zardooz, and M. Kamalnegad. 2004. Effects of *Papaver rhoeas* extract on the expression and development of morphine dependence in mice. *Journal of Ethnopharmacology* 95 (2–3): 431–5.

Soulimani, R., C. Younos, S. Jarmouni-Idrissi, D. Bousta, F. Khallouki, and A. Laila. 2001. Behavioral and pharmaco-toxicological study of *Papaver rhoeas* L. in mice. *Journal of Ethnopharmacology* 74 (3): 265–74.

ཆུ་སྲིན་སྡེར་མོ་

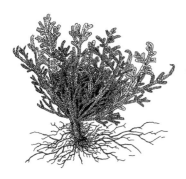

Wylie	*chu srin sder mo*
Drug name	Spike moss
Botanical name	*Selaginella doederleinii* or *S. tamariscina*
Part used	Entire plant
Taste and properties	Bitter and acrid; cooling

Traditional Actions and Clinical Uses

- Cools heat.
- Heals broken bones.
- Facilitates the flow of urine.
- Treats stomach and liver disorders.

Procurement

Spike moss is available from Chinese herbalists as *juan bai* (卷柏) or *shi shang bai* (石上柏).

Known Pharmacological Properties

Spike moss has anticancer properties (Bensky and Gamble 1986; Chinese Materia Medica 2002). It also has antiulcer, antibacterial, and hemostatic actions (Chinese Materia Medica 2002).

Herbs That Treat Contagious Diseases

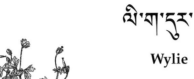

ལི་ག་དུར་

Wylie	*li ga dur*
Drug name	Cranesbill
Botanical name	*Geranium sp.*
Part used	Root
Taste and properties	Astringent, acrid, and sweet; cooling

Traditional Actions and Clinical Uses

- Treats epidemic diseases, lung fever, and fever that affects the blood, the channels, and the internal organs.
- Detoxifies.
- Relieves swelling of the limbs.

Procurement

Cranesbill is available from Western herbalists.

Known Pharmacological Properties

Cranesbill has astringent, antithrombotic, antiviral, and hypotensive actions (Willard 1991).

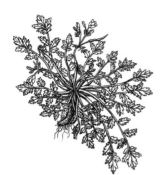

Wylie	*par pa ta*
Drug name	Fumitory
Botanical name	*Hypecoum leptocarpum*
Part used	Root, flower, and seed
Taste and properties	Bitter; cooling

Traditional Actions and Clinical Uses

- Treats toxic and epidemic fever: along with *gla sgang* (bistort), this is an important herb in the treatment of epidemic fever.
- Treats fever of the blood.
- Treats fever of the liver.
- Treats unripe fever.

Procurement and Variants

Fumitory is hard to find. Research for equivalent herbs could be made on the basis of its alkaloid profile.

Known Pharmacological Properties

Fumitory has choleretic, bronchodilatory, antibacterial, carotid vasodilatory, slight antitussive, and miotic actions. Its antibacterial action is caused by an increase in phagocytosis. It can lower intraocular pressure and thus may be helpful for glaucoma (Chinese Materia Medica 2002).

Additional References

Bentley, K. W. 1984. Beta-phenylethylamines and the isoquinoline alkaloids. *Natural Product Reports* 1 (4): 355–70.

Chen, B. Z., and Q. C. Fang. 1985. Chemical study on a traditional Tibetan drug *Hypecoum leptocarpum* (in Chinese). *Acta Pharmaceutica Sinica* 20 (9): 658–61.

Yi Zhou, Guolin Zhang, and Bogang Li. 1999. Five alkaloids from *Hypecoum leptocarpum*. *Phytochemistry* 50 (2): 339–43.

Zhang, G. L., G. Rucker, E. Breitmaier, and R. Mayer. 1995. Alkaloids from *Hypecoum leptocarpum*. *Phytochemistry* 40 (6): 1813–6.

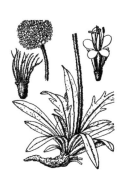

སྤང་རྩི་དོ་བོ་

Wylie	*spang rtsi do bo*
Botanical name	*Pterocephalus hookeri*
Part used	Entire plant
Taste and properties	Sweet and bitter; cooling

Traditional Actions and Clinical Uses

- Treats lung disorders, especially when there is pus.
- Treats infectious disorders, especially disturbed fever.

Procurement and Variants

This herb is hard to find outside of its habitat. It seems to be clinically and morphologically similar to dandelion.

དེ་ཐ་

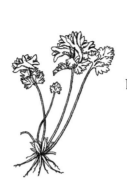

Wylie	*de wa*
Botanical name	*Corydalis melanochlora*
Part used	Entire plant
Taste and properties	Sweet and bitter; cooling

Traditional Actions and Clinical Uses

Treats infectious fever, bile fever, and fever in the channels.

Procurement and Variants

Willow *(shing 'byar pa)* may be used as a substitute for *shing de wa (Populus bonatii)*, another variety of *de wa* (Pasang Yonten Arya 1998). The bark is available from Western herbalists.

Herbs That Treat Phlegm

པི་པི་ལིང་

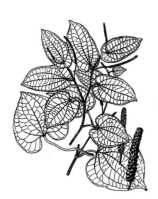

Wylie	*pi pi ling*
Drug name	Long pepper
Botanical name	*Piper longum*
Part used	Seed
Taste and properties	Sweet and pungent; warming, coarse, and sharp

Traditional Actions and Clinical Uses

- Treats all cold disorders, especially those associated with wind and phlegm with mucus, indigestion, and bloating.
- Restores kidney heat.
- Purifies the blood.
- Long pepper is also used in cooling formulas to protect the spleen from the damaging effects of cold herbs.

Procurement

Long pepper is available from Ayurvedic herbalists as *pippali* and from Chinese herbalists as *bi ba* (荜拔). It is also a common spice in Indian, African, and Indonesian cooking.

Known Pharmacological Properties

Long pepper has immunomodulatory, stimulant, antiasthmatic, anticancer, hepatoprotective, antiamoebic, antiulcer, hypolipidemic, anti-inflammatory, and antibiotic actions (Williamson 2002). When taken with black pepper and ginger, long pepper enhances the bioavailability of other herbs.

Additional References

C. K. Atal, Usha Zutshi, and P. G. Rao. 1981. Scientific evidence on the role of Ayurvedic herbals on bioavailability of drugs. *Journal of Ethnopharmacology* 4 (2): 229–32.

Hullatti, K. K., Uma D. Murthy, and B. R. Shrinath. 2006. In vitro and in vivo inhibitory effects of *Piper longum* fruit extracts on mouse Ehrlich ascites carcinoma. *Pharmacognosy Magazine* 2 (2): 220–3.

Khajuria, A., N. Thusu, and U. Zutshi. 2002. Piperine modulates permeability characteristics of intestine by inducing alterations in membrane dynamics: Influence on brush border membrane fluidity, ultra-structure, and enzyme kinetics. *Phytomedicine* 9(3): 224–31.

སེ་འབྲུ་

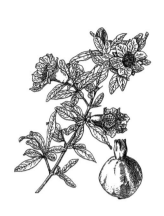

Wylie	*se 'bru*
Drug name	Pomegranate
Botanical name	*Punica granatum*
Part used	Dried seed and fruit
Taste and properties	Sour and sweet; warming and oily

Traditional Actions and Clinical Uses

- Treats stomach disorders, increases digestive heat, and improves digestion. Its seeds may be taken as a decoction on a regular basis (Thubten Phuntsog 2001).
- Treats diarrhea due to cold phlegm.
- Treats cold and wind disorders.

Procurement

Dried pomegranate seeds can be found whole and powdered at Indian grocery stores, where they are known as *anardana*.

Known Pharmacological Properties

Pomegranate seed has antibacterial, antioxidant, estrogenic, and uterine relaxant actions (Ross 1999). Antiangiogenic and anti-inflammatory actions have also been reported.

Additional References

Lansky, E. P., and R. A. Newman. (2007) *Punica granatum* (pomegranate) and its potential for prevention and treatment of inflammation and cancer. *Journal of Ethnopharmacology* 109 (2): 177–206.

Toi, M., H. Bando, C. Ramachandran, S. J. Melnick, A. Imai, R. S. Fife, R. E. Carr, T. Oikawa, and E. P. Lansky. 2003. Preliminary studies on the anti-angiogenic potential of pomegranate fractions in vitro and in vivo. *Angiogenesis* 6 (2): 121–8.

སུག་སྨེལ་

Wylie	*sug smel*
Drug name	Green cardamom
Botanical name	*Elettaria cardamomum*
Part used	Seed with or without shell
Taste and properties	Sweet, acrid, and slightly astringent; warming and sharp

Traditional Actions and Clinical Uses

Treats cold disorders, especially of the kidneys; increases digestive heat; and improves physical strength: this is one of the Six Excellent Drugs used in many formulas.

Procurement

Green cardamom is a common spice.

Known Pharmacological Properties

Green cardamom has anti-inflammatory, antispasmodic, and gastrostimulant actions (Caldecott 2006).

སྨན་སྒ་

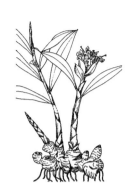

Wylie	*sman sga*
Drug name	Ginger
Botanical name	*Zingiber officinale*
Part used	Root
Taste and properties	Acrid, bitter, and astringent; warming

Traditional Actions and Clinical Uses

- Increases the appetite.
- Restores digestive heat.
- Treats wind and phlegm disorders.

Procurement and Variants

Fresh ginger (*bca' sga*) is a common foodstuff. It is considered interchangeable with dry ginger (*sman sga*), a common spice. Ginger may also be substituted with *sga skya* (galangal or spiked ginger lily) or *dong gra* (lesser galangal).

Known Pharmacological Properties

Ginger has antiemetic, antiulcer, hepatoprotective, anti-inflammatory, antiplatelet, antipyretic, hypolipidemic, antioxidant, immunomodulatory, thermogenic, anti-convulsant, antispasmodic, cardiotonic, anticancer, cholagogic, choleretic, digestant, hypoglycemic, antithrombotic, antinausea, and antiviral actions (Ross 1999; Williamson 2002). Antiangiogenesis has also been reported.

Additional References

Kim, E. C., J. K. Min, T. Y. Kim, S. J. Lee, H. O. Yang, S. Han, Y. M. Kim, and Y. G. Kwon. 2005. [6]-Gingerol, a pungent ingredient of ginger, inhibits angiogenesis in vitro and in vivo. *Biochemical and Biophysical Research Communications* 335 (2): 300–8.
Zingiber officinale (ginger) monograph. 2003. *Alternative Medicine Review* 8 (3): 331–5.

ཤིང་ཚ་

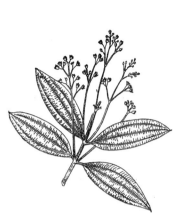

Wylie	*shing tsha*
Drug name	Cinnamon
Botanical name	*Cinnamomum aromaticum, C. cassia*, or *C. zeylanicum*
Part used	Bark
Taste and properties	Acrid, sweet, and astringent; warming, oily, and light

Traditional Actions and Clinical Uses

- Treats cold disorders and wind disorders of the liver and stomach.
- Restores digestive heat and improves digestion.

Procurement and Variants

Indian cinnamon is available from Ayurvedic herbalists as *tvak*. Common cinnamon is probably an adequate substitute.

Known Pharmacological Properties

Cinnamon has digestive, hypotensive, vasodilatory, leukopoietic, and antibacterial actions (Chang and But 1986). Hypoglycemic and immunomodulatory actions have been reported.

Additional References

Cao, H., M. M. Polansky, and R. A. Anderson. 2007. Cinnamon extract and polyphenols affect the expression of tristetraprolin, insulin receptor, and glucose transporter 4 in mouse 3T3-L1 adipocytes. *Archives of Biochemistry and Biophysics* 459 (2): 214–22.

Cao, H., J. F. Urban Jr., and R. A. Anderson. 2008. Cinnamon polyphenol extract affects immune responses by regulating anti- and proinflammatory and glucose transporter gene expression in mouse macrophages. *Journal of Nutrition* 138 (5): 833–40.

ན་ལེ་ཤམ་
ཕོ་བ་རིས་

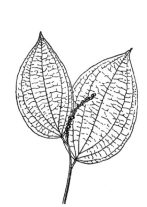

Wylie	*na le sham, pho ba ris*
Drug name	Black pepper
Botanical name	*Piper nigrum*
Part used	Fruit
Taste and properties	Acrid; warming

Traditional Actions and Clinical Uses

- Treats phlegm and cold disorders: this is an important herb in the treatment of phlegm. It is also used as an adjunct in the treatment of cold wind disorders.
- Improves the appetite.

Procurement

Black pepper is a common spice.

Known Pharmacological Properties

Black pepper has antimicrobial, anticancer, anti-inflammatory, antioxidant, and anticonvulsant actions. It also increases the secretion of stomach acid and of detoxifying liver enzymes (Williamson 2002). When taken with long pepper and ginger, black pepper enhances the bioavailability of other herbs. Potential antiulcer action has also been reported.

Additional References

Al-Moflehi, A., A. A. Alhaider, J. S. Mossa, M. O. Al-Sohaibani, S. Rafatullah, and S. Qureshi. 2005. Inhibition of gastric mucosal damage by *Piper nigrum* (black pepper) pretreatment in Wistar albino rats. *Pharmacognosy Magazine* 1 (2): 64–8.

Atal, C. K., Usha Zutshi, and P. G. Rao. 1981. Scientific evidence on the role of Ayurvedic herbals on bioavailability of drugs, *Journal of Ethnopharmacology* 4 (2): 229–32.

Khajuria, A., N. Thusu, and U. Zutshi. 2002. Piperine modulates permeability characteristics of intestine by inducing alterations in membrane dynamics: Influence on brush border membrane fluidity, ultra-structure and enzyme kinetics. *Phytomedicine* 9(3): 224–31.

ཀ་ཀོ་ལ་

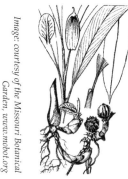

Image: courtesy of the Missouri Botanical Garden, www.mobot.org

Wylie	*ka ko la*
Drug name	Black cardamom
Botanical name	*Amomum subulatum*
Part used	Seed
Taste and properties	Sweet and acrid; warming and light

Traditional Actions and Clinical Uses

Treats poor digestion: this is one of the Six Excellent Drugs used in many formulas.

Procurement

Black cardamom is a common Indian spice.

Known Pharmacological Properties

Black cardamom has antiulcer and antioxidant actions.

References

Dhuley, J. N. 1999. Antioxidant effects of cinnamon (*Cinnamomum verum*) bark and greater cardamom (*Amomum subulatum*) seeds in rats fed high fat diet. *Indian journal of experimental biology* 37 (3): 238–42.

Jafri, M. A., Farah, K. Javed, and S. Singh. 2001. Evaluation of the gastric antiulcerogenic effect of large cardamom (fruits of *Amomum subulatum* Roxb.). *Journal of Ethnopharmacology* 75 (2–3): 89–94.

Kikuzaki, H., Y. Kawai, and N. Nakatani. 2001. 1,1-Diphenyl-2-picrylhydrazyl radical-scavenging active compounds from greater cardamom (*Amomum subulatum* Roxb.). *Journal of Nutritional Science and Vitaminology* 47 (2): 167–71.

Owen, P. L., and T. Johns. 2002. Antioxidants in medicines and spices as cardioprotective agents in Tibetan highlanders. *Pharmaceutical Biology* 40 (5): 346–57.

Yadav, A. S., and D. Bhatnagar. 2007. Modulatory effect of spice extracts on iron-induced lipid peroxidation in rat liver. *BioFactors* 29 (2–3): 147–57.

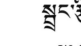

Wylie	*sbrang rtsi*
Drug name	Honey
Latin name	*Mel apis*
Taste and properties	Sweet; warming

Traditional Actions and Clinical Uses

Serves as a vehicle for preparations used to treat phlegm and lymph *(chu ser)* disorders.

Procurement

Honey is a common foodstuff.

Known Pharmacological Properties

Honey has an antibacterial action. It alleviates diarrhea by slowing peristalsis. It has no demonstrated hypoglycemic or hyperglycemic action. It is useful in aconite poisoning, can help weight gain, and aids regeneration of the liver (Chinese Materia Medica 2002).

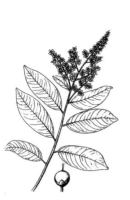

བྱི་ཏང་ག་

Wylie	*byi tang ga*
Drug name	False black pepper
Botanical name	*Embelia ribes*
Part used	Fruit
Taste and properties	Sweet and sour; warming

Traditional Actions and Clinical Uses

- Increases digestive heat: false black pepper is used in the treatment of phlegm.
- Expels parasites.

Procurement

False black pepper is available from Ayurvedic herbalists as *vidanga*.

Known Pharmacological Properties

False black pepper has anthelmintic, analgesic, hypoglycemic, antitumor, and antimicrobial actions. It also has contraceptive effects in both male and female mammals and in women (Caldecott 2006; Williamson 2002).

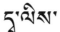

Wylie	*dwa lis*
Drug name	Rhododendron
Botanical name	*Rhododendron anthopogonoides*
Part used	Leaf and flower
Taste and properties	Bitter and astringent; warming

Traditional Actions and Clinical Uses

- Treats cold phlegm and restores digestive heat.
- Benefits the lungs.
- Treats diseases caused by hot or cold climate.

Procurement and Variants

The Chinese variety *(Rhododendron molle)* is sometimes available as *nao yang hua* (闹羊花).

Known Pharmacological Properties

Chinese rhododendron has hypotensive, bradycardic, analgesic, and smooth-muscle stimulant actions (Chang and But 1987).

ཨེ་ར་དཀར་པོ་

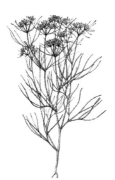

Wylie	*zi ra dkar po*
Drug name	Cumin
Botanical name	*Cuminum cyminum*
Part used	Seed
Taste and properties	Acrid and sweet; warming

Traditional Actions and Clinical Uses

- Increases digestive heat.
- Improves the appetite.

Procurement

Cumin is a common spice.

Known Pharmacological Properties

Cumin has antimicrobial, antithrombotic, and estrogenic actions. It has a dose-dependent action on the metabolism of pharmaceuticals (Gruenwald et al. 2000). Cumin essential oil can enhance morphine dependence and tolerance and has hypoglycemic, antitumor, gastrostimulant, hypolipidemic, antiepileptic, and antioxidant actions. Cumin can enhance the bioavailability of pharmaceuticals. A protective effect against 1,2-dimethylhydrazine-induced colon cancer was found. Cumin has a protective effect against the toxicity of alcohol and heat-oxidized sunflower oil, a powerful carcinogen.

Additional References

Aruna, K., R. Rukkumani, P. S. Varma, and V. P. Menon. 2005. Therapeutic role of *Cuminum cyminum* on ethanol and thermally oxidized sunflower oil induced toxicity. *Phytotherapy Research* 19 (5): 416–21.

Dhandapani, S., V. R. Subramanian, S. Rajagopal, and N. Namasivayam. 2002. Hypolipidemic effect of *Cuminum cyminum* L. on alloxan-induced diabetic rats. *Pharmacological Research* 46 (3): 251–5.

Gagandeep, S. Dhanalakshmi, E. Méndiz, A. R. Rao, and R. K. Kale. 2003. Chemopreventive effects of *Cuminum cyminum* in chemically induced forestomach and uterine cervix tumors in murine model systems. *Nutrition and Cancer* 47 (2): 171–80.

Haghparast, A., J. Shams, A. Khatibi, A. M. Alizadeh, and M. Kamalinejad. 2008. Effects of the fruit essential oil of *Cuminum cyminum* Linn. (Apiaceae) on acquisition and expression of morphine tolerance and dependence in mice. *Neuroscience Letters* 440 (2): 134–9.

Iacobellis, N. S., P. Lo Cantore, F. Capasso, and F. Senatore. 2005. Antibacterial activity of *Cuminum cyminum* L. and *Carum carvi* L. essential oils. *Journal of Agricultural and Food Chemistry* 53 (1): 57–61.

Janahmadi, M., F. Niazi, S. Danyali, and M. Kamalinejad. 2006. Effects of the fruit essential oil of *Cuminum cyminum* Linn. (Apiaceae) on pentylenetetrazol-induced epileptiform activity in F1 neurones of *Helix aspersa*. *Journal of Ethnopharmacology* 104 (1–2): 278–82.

Nalini, N., V. Manju, and V. P. Menon. 2006. Effect of spices on lipid metabolism in 1,2-dimethylhydrazine-induced rat colon carcinogenesis. *Journal of Medicinal Food* 9 (2): 237–45.

Sachin, B. S., S. C. Sharma, S. Sethi, S. A. Tasduq, M. K. Tikoo, A. K. Tikoo, N. K. Satti, B. D. Gupta, K. A. Suri, R. K. Johri, and G. N. Qazi. 2007. Herbal modulation of drug bioavailability: Enhancement of rifampicin levels in plasma by herbal products and a flavonoid glycoside derived from *Cuminum cyminum*. *Phytotherapy Research* 21 (2): 157–63.

Satyanarayana, S., K. Sushruta, G. S. Sarma, N. Srinivas, and G. V. Subba Raju. 2004. Antioxidant activity of the aqueous extracts of spicy food additives—evaluation and comparison with ascorbic acid in in-vitro systems. *Journal of Herbal Pharmacotherapy* 4 (2): 1–10.

Srinivasan, K. 2005. Plant foods in the management of diabetes mellitus: Spices as beneficial antidiabetic food adjuncts. *International Journal of Food Sciences and Nutrition* 56 (6): 399–414.

Topal, U., M. Sasaki, M. Goto, and S. Otles. 2007. Chemical compositions and antioxidant properties of essential oils from nine species of Turkish plants obtained by supercritical carbon dioxide extraction and steam distillation. *International Journal of Food Sciences and Nutrition* 18: 1–16.

Vasudevan, K., S. Vembar, K. Veeraraghavan, and P. S. Haranath. 2000. Influence of intragastric perfusion of aqueous spice extracts on acid secretion in anesthetized albino rats. *Indian journal of Gastroenterology* 19 (2): 53–6.

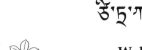

ཙི་ཏྲ་ཀ་

Wylie	*tsi tra ka*
Drug name	Wild leadwort
Botanical name	*Plumbago zeylanica*
Part used	Fruit
Taste and properties	Acrid; extremely warming

Traditional Actions and Clinical Uses

Increases digestive heat with fire-like power.

Procurement

Wild leadwort is available from Ayurvedic herbalists as *chitrak*.

Known Pharmacological Properties

Wild leadwort has anticancer, antifertility, anti-inflammatory, antimicrobial, antioxidant, immunomodulatory, hypolipidemic, uterotonic, and anticoagulant actions (Williamson 2002). Plumbagin, a constituent of wild leadwort, prevented the development of antibiotic resistance of *Escherichia coli* and *Staphylococcus aureus* in vitro. The root of the plant stimulated the proliferation of coliform bacteria in mice, thus normalizing their intestinal flora.

Additional References

Durga, R., P. Sridhar, and H. Polasa. 1990. Effects of plumbagin on antibiotic resistance in bacteria. *Indian Journal of Medical Research* 91 (A): 18–20.

Iyengar, M. A., and G. S. Pendse. 1966. *Plumbago zeylanica* L. (Chitrak), a gastrointestinal flora normaliser. *Planta Medica* 14 (3): 337–51.

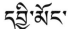

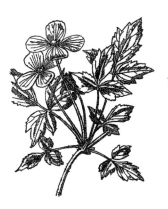

Wylie	*dbyi mong*
Drug name	Clematis
Botanical name	*Clematis montana* or *C. tibetana*
Part used	Stem, leaf, flower, and seed
Taste and properties	Acrid and slightly sweet; warming, light, sharp, and coarse

Traditional Actions and Clinical Uses

- Restores digestive heat.
- Treats diarrhea caused by impaired digestion.
- Dries serous fluid.
- Treats infectious diseases.
- Reduces tumors due to cold in the large intestine.

Procurement and Variants

A closely related species, *Clematis armandii*, is sometimes sold by Chinese herbalists as *chuan mu tong* (川木通). However, the United States Food and Drug Administration determined that both this species and *Clematis montana* contains aristolochic acid, a dangerous nephrotoxin. The status of *Clematis tibetana* is unclear.

Known Pharmacological Properties

Clematis has diuretic action and can especially help eliminate sodium (Chinese Materia Medica 2002).

ད་ཏྲིག་

Wylie	*da trig*
Drug name	Schisandra
Botanical name	*Schisandra chinensis*
Part used	Fruit
Taste and properties	Sweet and sour; neutral

Traditional Actions and Clinical Uses

- Checks vomiting, diarrhea, excessive perspiration, and loss of reproductive fluids and improves the appetite: schisandra is used in the treatment of phlegm and especially dark phlegm.
- Benefits the lungs.

Procurement

Schisandra can be obtained from Chinese herbalists as *wu wei zi* (五味子).

Known Pharmacological Properties

Schisandra has CNS stimulant, antistress, endurance-enhancing, respiratory stimulant, anti-inflammatory, antiulcer, hypotensive, expectorant, antioxidant, antitumor, hepatoprotective, uterotonic, vasodilator, hyperglycemic, adaptogenic, and antibacterial actions (Chang and But 1986; WHO 2007).

ཟི་ར་ནག་པོ་

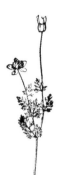

Wylie	*zi ra nag po*
Drug name	Fennelflower
Botanical name	*Nigella glandulifera*
Part used	Seed
Taste and properties	Sweet; warming and oily

Traditional Actions and Clinical Uses

- Treats stomach disorders.
- Treats cold liver disorders.

Procurement

The Indian variety *(Nigella sativa)* is probably an adequate substitute. It is available at Indian grocery stores, where it is called *kalonji* or (incorrectly) black onion seed.

Known Pharmacological Properties

The Indian variety *(Nigella sativa)* has antimicrobial, hepatoprotective, hypo-glycemic, anti-inflammatory, cytotoxic, anthelmintic, analgesic, and other actions (Williamson 2002).

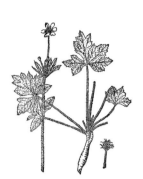

 སྲུབ་ཀ་

Wylie	*srub ka*
Botanical name	*Anemone rivularis*
Part used	Seed
Taste and properties	Astringent and very acrid; warming

Traditional Actions and Clinical Uses

- Restores bodily heat and digestive heat.
- Relieves pain.
- Dries serous fluid.
- Treats cold tumors.

Procurement

Anemone rivularis is known to Chinese botanists as *cao wu mei* (草玉梅), but its availability as a medicinal is uncertain.

ম་རུ་རྩེ

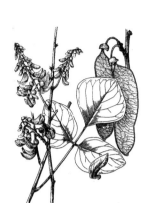

Wylie	*ma ru rtse*
Drug name	Flame of the forest
Botanical name	*Butea frondosa* syn. *B. monosperma*
Part used	Fruit
Taste and properties	Bitter and sweet

Traditional Actions and Clinical Uses

- Treats phlegm and arthritis.
- Expels parasites.

Procurement

Flame of the forest fruit may be available from Ayurvedic sources as *palasa* or *palasha*.

Known Pharmacological Properties

Flame of the forest can help prevent miscarriage by inhibiting the decidual cells of the uterus. It also has an antiparasitic action (Chinese Materia Medica 2002).

རོང་ག྄་

Wylie	*dong gra*
Drug name	Lesser galangal
Botanical name	*Alpinia officinarum*
Part used	Root
Taste and properties	Acrid; warming

Traditional Actions and Clinical Uses

- Increases body heat.
- Improves the appetite.
- Removes pus from the lungs.

Procurement

Lesser galangal is available from Chinese herbalists as *gao liang jiang* (高良姜).

Known Pharmacological Properties

Lesser galangal has an antibiotic action and can stimulate or inhibit guinea-pig intestines depending on dosage (Bensky and Gamble 1986).

བུལ་ཏོག་

Wylie	*bul tog*
Drug name	Soda ash
Taste and properties	Bitter and salty; warming

Traditional Actions and Clinical Uses

- Stops necrosis due to internal injury.
- Helps promote the digestion of grain.
- Treats poisoning.

Chemical Composition

Sodium carbonate, Na_2CO_3

Procurement

Soda ash is available from chemical suppliers.

Herbs That Treat Phlegm and Wind

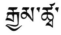

Wylie	*rgyam tshwa*
Drug name	Rock salt
Latin name	*Sal*
Taste and properties	Salty and slightly sweet; warming

Traditional Actions and Clinical Uses

- Treats indigestion.
- Treats phlegm disorders.
- Treats wind disorders.

Chemical Composition

Sodium chloride, trace elements

Procurement

Table salt is suitable. Anticaking agents such as aluminum hydroxide, sodium ferrocyanide, etc. should be avoided.

ब्र་སྐྱ་

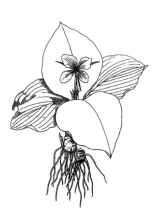

Wylie	*sga skya*
Drug name	Galangal or spiked ginger lily
Botanical name	*Kaempferia galanga* or *Hedychium spicatum*
Part used	Root
Taste and properties	Acrid and astringent; warming and sharp

Traditional Actions and Clinical Uses

- Treats wind and phlegm.
- Restores digestive heat.
- Helps the circulation of blood.

Procurement and Variants

Galangal is a common spice in Asia. There exist several varieties of galangal *(Kaempferia galanga)*, all of which probably have similar effects.

Known Pharmacological Properties

Galangal has anticancer, vasorelaxant, anti-*Helicobacter,* antioxidant, vulnerary, antimicrobial, and anti-inflammatory actions.

References

Bhamarapravati, S., S. L. Pendland, and G. B. Mahady. 2003. Extracts of spice and food plants from Thai traditional medicine inhibit the growth of the human carcinogen *Helicobacter pylori. In Vivo* 17 (6): 541–4.

Chen, I. N., C. C. Chang, C. C. Ng, C. Y. Wang, Y. T. Shyu, and T. L. Chang. 2008. Antioxidant and antimicrobial activity of Zingiberaceae plants in Taiwan. *Plant Foods for Human Nutrition* 63 (1): 15–20.

Chirangini, P., G. J. Sharma, and S. K. Sinha. 2004. Sulfur free radical reactivity with curcumin as reference for evaluating antioxidant properties of medicinal zingiberales. *Journal of Environmental Pathology, Toxicology and Oncology* 23 (3): 227–36.

Othman, R., H. Ibrahim, M. A. Mohd, K. Awang, A. U. Gilani, and M. R. Mustafa. 2002. Vasorelaxant effects of ethyl cinnamate isolated from *Kaempferia galanga* on smooth muscles of the rat aorta. *Planta Medica* 68 (7): 655–7, and subsequent articles by the same authors.

Tara Shanbhag, V., S. Chandrakala, A. Sachidananda, B. L. Kurady, S. Smita, and S. Ganesh. 2006. Wound healing activity of alcoholic extract of *Kaempferia galanga* in Wistar rats. *Indian Journal of Physiology and Pharmacology* 50 (4): 384–90.

Vimala, S., A. W. Norhanom, and M. Yadav. 1999. Anti-tumour promoter activity in Malaysian ginger rhizobia used in traditional medicine. *British Journal of Cancer* 80 (1–2): 110–6.

Xue, Y., and H. Chen. 2002. Study on the anti-carcinogenic effects of three compounds in *Kaempferia galanga* L. *Journal of Hygiene Research* (China; article in Chinese) 31 (4): 247–8, 251.

ཁ་རུ་ཚྭ་

Wylie	*kha ru tshwa*
Drug name	Black salt
Latin name	*Halitum violaceum*
Taste and properties	Acrid and salty; warming and oily

Traditional Actions and Clinical Uses

- Increases digestive heat: this is an important remedy for impaired digestion. It may be added to foods to help digestion (Tibetan Medicine Program 2007).
- Treats phlegm in the upper part of the body.
- Treats wind in the lower part of the body.

Chemical Composition

Sodium chloride and trace amounts of potassium, calcium, iron, aluminum, titanium, manganese, barium, magnesium, strontium, copper, sulfur, and silicon (Chinese Materia Medica 2002)

Procurement

Black salt is available from Indian grocery stores.

Known Pharmacological Properties

Black salt has an anticancer action in rats that seems related to the metabolism of sulfur, iron, calcium, and selenium (Chinese Materia Medica 2002).

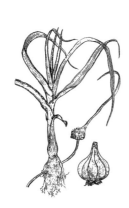

ষ্গོག་སྐྱ་

Wylie	*sgog skya*
Drug name	Garlic
Botanical name	*Allium sativum*
Part used	Root
Taste and properties	Acrid; warming, heavy, sharp, and oily

Traditional Actions and Clinical Uses

- Treats wind, especially in a broth combined with bones and *bu ram* (raw cane sugar).
- Treats fever associated with wind.
- Restores digestive heat and improves appetite, but may cause sleepiness.
- Expels parasites.

Procurement

Garlic is a common foodstuff.

Known Pharmacological Properties

Garlic has numerous beneficial effects, including immunomodulatory, antiaging, hypolipidemic, hepatoprotective, antibiotic, antiviral, antioxidant, anticancer, diuretic, antiplatelet, and hypotensive actions (Ross 1999; Williamson 2002).

Herbs That Treat Phlegm Disorders Associated with Heat

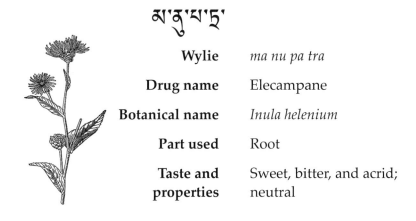

མ་ནུ་པ་ཏ་

Wylie	*ma nu pa tra*
Drug name	Elecampane
Botanical name	*Inula helenium*
Part used	Root
Taste and properties	Sweet, bitter, and acrid; neutral

Traditional Actions and Clinical Uses

- Treats combined blood and wind disorders and combined bile and phlegm disorders: elecampane is mentioned in the Oral Instruction Tantra in the treatment of dark phlegm and other disorders.
- Restores digestive heat.
- Treats epidemic fever of recent origin: elecampane is often used in combination with *sle tres* (moonseed), *kaNDa ka ri* (two-flowered raspberry), and *sga skya* (galangal) to treat recently acquired fever, to gather or ripen fever, or to make hidden fever manifest.

Procurement

Elecampane is available from Chinese herbalists as *tu mu xiang* (土木香) and from Western herbalists. A closely-related species, *pu Shkara mU la (Inula racemosa)*, is available from Ayurvedic herbalists as *pushkarmool.*

Known Pharmacological Properties

Elecampane has insecticidal, antibacterial, and antifungal actions. It slows intestinal secretions and peristalsis. It relieves pain and lowers the effect of fatigue in skeletal muscles. It has a vasodilatory action in small doses and a vasoconstrictor action in large doses (Chinese Materia Medica 2002). It also has an anticancer action.

Additional Reference

Goun, E. A., V. M. Petrichenko, S. U. Solodnikov, T. V. Suhinina, M. A. Kline, G. Cunningham, C. Nguyen, and H. Miles. 2002. Anticancer and antithrombin activity of Russian plants. *Journal of Ethnopharmacology* 81 (3): 337–42.

ཨུ་སུ་

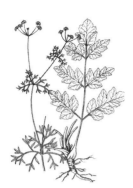

Wylie	*'u su*
Drug name	Coriander
Botanical name	*Coriandrum sativum*
Part used	Seed
Taste and properties	Sweet, acrid, and slightly bitter; warming, oily, and light

Traditional Actions and Clinical Uses

- Restores digestive heat.
- Treats phlegm.
- Treats dark phlegm.
- Relieves abdominal spasms.

Procurement

Coriander is a common spice.

Known Pharmacological Properties

Coriander seed has an antioxidant action and increases vitamin-A absorption but reduces the intestinal absorption of choline (Chinese Materia Medica 2002).

ཕྱི་ཡང་ཀུ་

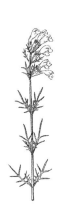

Wylie	*pri yang ku*
Drug name	Nodding dragonhead
Botanical name	*Dracocephalum tanguticum*
Part used	Aerial part of the plant
Taste and properties	Sweet and bitter; cooling

Traditional Actions and Clinical Uses

- Treats hot liver and stomach disorders.
- Treats dark phlegm.
- Treats water retention due to heat.

Procurement

Nodding dragonhead seeds are available from seed vendors.

Known Pharmacological Properties

Nodding dragonhead improves the blood's oxygen binding capacity and protects the lungs, liver, and kidneys against hypoxia (Chinese Materia Medica 2002).

Additional Reference

Hai, P., S. Zhou, H. Shang, and G. Zhao. 1997. Antianoxic effects of *Dracocephalum tanguticum* on brain of mice. *Journal of Chinese Medicinal Materials* (in Chinese) 20 (4): 198–200.

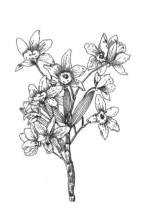

ཕུ་ཤེལ་རྩེ་

Wylie	*pu shel rtse*
Drug name	Noble dendrobium
Botanical name	*Dendrobium sp.*
Part used	Stems
Taste and properties	Sweet; cooling, light

Traditional Actions and Clinical Uses

- Treats vomiting.
- Quenches thirst.
- Lowers fever associated with phlegm.
- Restores the power of digestion.
- Noble dendrobium is mentioned in the Oral Instruction Tantra in the treatment of dark phlegm.

Procurement and Variants

Noble dendrobium is available from Chinese herbalists as various *Dendrobium* species sold under the common drug name *shi hu* (石斛). The species *Dendrobium officinale* and *Dendrobium wilsonii* are threatened (IUCN 2009), but a number of closely related species may be of lesser concern, including *Dendrobium nobile*. The suitability of other *Dendrobium* species to Tibetan medicine must be verified.

Known Pharmacological Properties

Noble dendrobium has analgesic, antipyretic, and heart-relaxant actions (Bensky and Gamble 1986). It has anti-inflammatory, anticancer, hypoglycemic, uterotonic, and vasodilatory actions, increases phagocytosis, and prevents cataract in rats' eyes by lowering cholesterol (Chinese Materia Medica 2002).

བསེ་ཡབ་

Wylie	*bse yab*
Drug name	Chinese quince
Botanical name	*Chaenomeles lagenaria*
Part used	Fruit
Taste and properties	Sour and sweet; cooling

Traditional Actions and Clinical Uses

- Treats dark phlegm.
- Treats chronic hot stomach disorders.

Procurement

Chinese quince is available from Chinese herbalists as *mu gua* (木瓜).

Known Pharmacological Properties

Chinese quince has an anti-inflammatory action (Bensky and Gamble 1986). It also has hepatoprotective and antibacterial actions (Chinese Materia Medica 2002).

Wylie	*sbrul gyi sha*
Drug name	Processed snake meat
Taste and properties	Sweet, salty

Traditional Actions and Clinical Uses

- Regulates the menses and facilitates childbirth.
- Treats dark phlegm. Snake meat is used in the treatment of dark phlegm in combination with *star bu* (sea buckthorn), *rgyam tshwa* (rock salt), and other minerals and salts to help break up blood tumors.
- Benefits the liver and the eyes.

ཁུར་མང་

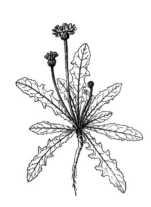

Wylie	*khur mang*
Drug name	Dandelion
Botanical name	*Taraxacum sp.*
Part used	Entire plant
Taste and properties	Bitter and slightly sweet; cooling

Traditional Actions and Clinical Uses

- Treats dark phlegm.
- Treats chronic fever, especially when it has penetrated the bones.
- Treats bile and toxins.

Procurement and Variants

The entire plant is available from Chinese herbalists as *pu gong ying* (蒲公英). Dandelion root and leaf are available separately from Western herbalists.

Known Pharmacological Properties

Dandelion has antimicrobial, laxative, immunostimulant, choleretic, hepatoprotective, stomachic, anti-inflammatory, antiulcer, hypoglycemic (the leaf only), and diuretic actions (Chang and But 1987; WHO 2007).

ཕག་ཁྲག་

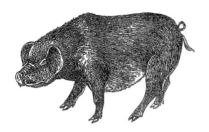

Wylie	*phag khrag*
Drug name	Pig's blood
Latin name	*Sus scrofa domestica*
Taste and properties	Sweet; cooling

Traditional Actions and Clinical Uses

Removes toxins and dark phlegm that have spread throughout the body.

Procurement and Variants

Pig's blood may be available at larger Chinese grocery stores.

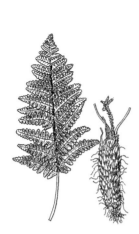

ཕུར་བུ་རེ་རལ་

Wylie	*ldum bu re ral*
Drug name	Fern
Botanical name	*Dryopteris sp.* or *Polystichum sp.*
Part used	Root
Taste and properties	Sweet and astringent; cooling, coarse, light, and slightly poisonous

Traditional Actions and Clinical Uses

- Treats meat poisoning and compounded poisoning.
- Treats dysentery.

Procurement and Variants

Male fern *(Dryopteris filix-mas)* is available from Western herbalists. A Chinese variety *(Dryopteris crassirhizoma)* is available from Chinese herbalists as *guan zhong* (贯众).

Known Pharmacological Properties

Chinese fern has a strong antiviral action and anthelmintic, uterotonic, abortifacient, estrogenic, hemostatic, heart inhibiting, and smooth-muscle actions (Chang and But 1987).

Emetics and Purgatives

 དུར་བྱིད་

Wylie	*dur byid*
Drug name	Spurge
Botanical name	*Euphorbia fischeriana* or *E. himalayensis*
Part used	Root
Taste and properties	Acrid; very warming, rough, and sharp

Traditional Actions and Clinical Uses

- Treats indigestion and stomach disorders.
- Evacuates feces: spurge is used in purgative formulas in the treatment of fever, bile, epidemic fever, phlegm, and dark-phlegm disorders.

Procurement and Variants

A Chinese variety of spurge is available from Chinese herbalists as *da ji* (大戟).

Known Pharmacological Properties

Spurge has cathartic and hypotensive actions but no demonstrated diuretic action (Bensky and Gamble 1986).

Remark

In traditional Chinese medicine, spurge is considered incompatible with *shing mngar* (licorice). This incompatibility has been verified by modern research (Bensky and Gamble 1986).

ལྕུམ་རྩ་

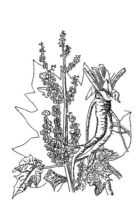

Wylie	*lcum rtsa*
Drug name	Rhubarb
Botanical name	*Rheum palmatum*
Part used	Root
Taste and properties	Sour; neutral and coarse

Traditional Actions and Clinical Uses

- Purges phlegm: rhubarb is used as a purgative in the treatment of phlegm and various hot disorders.
- Treats hot stomach disorders.
- Treats toxic fever.

Procurement

Rhubarb is available from Chinese herbalists as *da huang* (大黃).

Known Pharmacological Properties

Rhubarb has cathartic or antidiarrheal action depending on dosage and the way it is combined with other herbs. It is also antispasmodic, antibacterial, antifungal, antiviral, antiamoebic, diuretic, antineoplastic, hypotensive, hemostatic, antispasmodic, and choleretic, and it stimulates the appetite (Chang and But 1986).

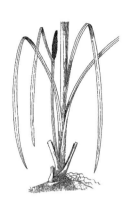

ཤུ་དག་

Wylie	*shu dag*
Drug name	Sweet flag
Botanical name	*Acorus calamus*
Part used	Root
Taste and properties	Bitter and acrid; warming and sharp

Traditional Actions and Clinical Uses

- Restores digestive heat.
- Balances the bodily constituents.
- Treats wind disorders, especially amnesia.
- Treats contagious fever.
- Treats wind that affects the heart.

Procurement and Variants

Tibetan medicine knows two varieties of sweet flag. *Acorus calamus (shu dag nag po)* is more common and contains less beta-asarone, a controversial chemical. It is available from Ayurvedic herbalists as *vacha* as well as from Western herbalists. *Acorus gramineus* or Japanese sweet flag *(shu dag dkar po)* is available from Chinese herbalists as *shi chang pu* (石菖蒲).

Known Pharmacological Properties

Sweet flag has antiulcer, antispasmodic, analgesic, CNS-depressant, neuroprotective, hypolipidemic, anti-inflammatory, anticonvulsant, and antibacterial actions (Caldecott 2006; Williamson 2002). Antiarrhythmic, hypotensive, antitussive, expectorant, and antiasthmatic actions were reported (Chang and But 1986, 282–8). Anticancer activity was reported.

Additional Reference

Goun, E. A., V. M. Petrichenko, S. U. Solodnikov, T. V. Suhinina, M. A. Kline, G. Cunningham, C. Nguyen, and H. Miles. 2002. Anticancer and antithrombin activity of Russian plants. *Journal of Ethnopharmacology* 81 (3): 337–42.

Herbs That Treat Poisoning

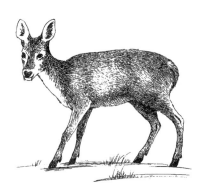

ग་རྩི

Wylie	*gla rtsi*
Drug name	Musk
Latin name	*Moschus moschiferus*
Part used	Secretion of the musk deer
Taste and properties	Acrid; cooling

Traditional Actions and Clinical Uses

- Treats poisoning.
- Expels worms.
- Treats disorders of the kidneys and liver.
- Treats infections.
- Treats eye and channel disorders.
- Treats urinary retention.
- Treats diseases caused by spirits.

Procurement and Variants

Since musk deer is endangered, most available musk is synthetic. However, not all commercial synthetic musk corresponds to the main constituents of deer musk, which are muscone and normuscone.

Known Pharmacological Properties

Musk increases heart contractions, diminishes the latency of conditioned reflexes, and increases beta-adrenergic responses. It has uterotonic, antibacterial, androgenic, anticancer, and strong anti-inflammatory actions. Metabolic research also suggests a stimulating action on liver enzymes and an increase in plasma cyclic AMP production (Chang and But 1987).

བསེ་རུའི་ར་

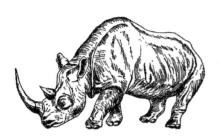

Wylie	*bse ru'i rwa*
Drug name	Rhinoceros horn
Latin name	*Rhinoceros sp.*
Part used	Horn
Taste and properties	Acrid and bitter; cooling

Traditional Actions and Clinical Uses

• Removes pus, blood, and lymph *(chu ser)* from the lungs and upper abdomen.
• Treats toxic fever.

Procurement and Variants

Rhinoceros is endangered. Well appreciated in Chinese medicine, rhinoceros horn has in recent times been substituted with the horn of the water buffalo, *shui niu jiao* (水牛角), in doses about twenty times larger. Most researchers believe that the horns of both animals are basically equivalent (Bensky and Gamble 1986; Chang and But 1987).

Known Pharmacological Properties

Both rhinoceros horn and water buffalo horn have cardiotonic, leukopoietic, and tranquilizing actions but no demonstrated antipyretic effect (Chang and But 1987).

ङ्गग་ཤ་

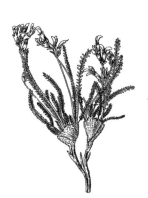

Wylie	*stag sha*
Drug name	Locoweed
Botanical name	*Oxytropis microphylla*
Part used	Leaf
Taste and properties	Bitter; cooling, and very poisonous

Traditional Actions and Clinical Uses

- Treats infectious fever.
- Treats lymph *(chu ser)* disorders.
- Reduces swelling.
- Stops bleeding.
- Detoxifies.
- Heals wounds and broken bones.

Known Pharmacological Properties

Locoweed has expectorant, slight bronchodilatory, antiarthritic, tachycardic, and hypertensive actions. The drug tends to accumulate in the kidneys, brain, and liver. Overdose causes arrhythmia with T-wave reversal, which resolves itself when the drug is discontinued (Chinese Materia Medica 2002).

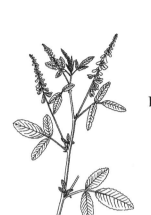

རྒྱ་སྤོས་

Wylie	*rgya spos*
Drug name	Clover
Botanical name	*Melilotus officinalis, M. suaveolens,* or *Trifolium pratense*
Part used	Entire plant
Taste and properties	Bitter; cooling

Traditional Actions and Clinical Uses

- Treats chronic fever.
- Treats toxic fever.
- Relieves abdominal spasms.

Procurement and Variants

Clover blossoms are available from Western herbalists.

Known Pharmacological Properties

Clover has antimalarial action (Chinese Materia Medica 2002). It has antispasmodic and expectorant actions and promotes the healing of skin (Gruenwald et al. 2000). It also has estrogenic and HDL-cholesterol boosting actions and can prevent bone loss in menopausal women. Beneficial action on benign and malignant prostate disorders has also been reported. In one study, a component of clover was found to lower LDL-C cholesterol in men but not in women.

Additional References

Atkinson, C., R. M. Warren, E. Sala, M. Dowsett, A. M. Dunning, C. S. Healey, S. Runswick, N. E. Day, and S. A. Bingham. 2004. Red-clover-derived isoflavones and mammographic breast density: A double-blind, randomized, placebo-controlled trial [ISRCTN42940165]. *Breast Cancer Research* 6 (3): R170–9.

Blakesmith, S. J., P. M. Lyons-Wall, C. George, G. E. Joannou, P. Petocz, and S. Samman. 2003. Effects of supplementation with purified red clover (*Trifolium pratense*) isoflavones on plasma lipids and insulin resistance in healthy premenopausal women. *British Journal of Nutrition* 89 (4): 467–74.

Booth N. L., C. E. Piersen, S. Banuvar, S. E. Geller, L. P. Shulman, and N. R. Farnsworth. 2006. Clinical studies of red clover (*Trifolium pratense*) dietary supplements in menopause: A literature review. *Menopause* 13 (2): 251–64.

Clifton-Bligh, P. B., R. J. Baber, G. R. Fulcher, M. L. Nery, and T. Moreton. 2001. The effect of isoflavones extracted from red clover (Rimostil) on lipid and bone metabolism. *Menopause* 8 (4): 259–65.

Griffiths, K., L. Denis, A. Turkes, and M. S. Morton. 1998. Phytoestrogens and diseases of the prostate gland. *Baillière's Clinical Endocrinology and Metabolism* 12 (4): 625–47.

Jarred, R. A., M. Keikha, C. Dowling, S. J. McPherson, A. M. Clare, A. J. Husband, J. S. Pedersen, M. Frydenberg, and G. P. Risbridger. 2002. Induction of apoptosis in low to moderate-grade human prostate carcinoma by red clover-derived dietary isoflavones. *Cancer Epidemiology, Biomarkers and Prevention* 11 (12): 1689–96.

Lam, A. N., M. Demasi, M. J. James, A. J. Husband, and C. Walker. 2004. Effect of red clover isoflavones on cox-2 activity in murine and human monocyte/macrophage cells. *Nutrition and Cancer* 49 (1): 89–93.

Nestel, P., M. Cehun, A. Chronopoulos, L. DaSilva, H. Teede, and B. McGrath. 2004. A biochanin-enriched isoflavone from red clover lowers LDL cholesterol in men. *European Journal of Clinical Nutrition* 58 (3): 403–8.

རྡོ་དྲེག་དམར་པོ་

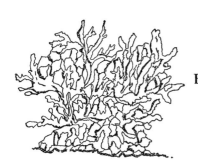

Wylie	*rdo dreg*
Drug name	Salted shield
Botanical name	*Parmelia saxatilis*
Part used	Entire plant
Taste and properties	Acrid; cooling, and slightly poisonous

Traditional Actions and Clinical Uses

Treats poisoning and chronic fever.

Procurement and Variants

Salted shield is a lichen that grows on rocks. In the commercial formulation Padma 28 or Padma Basic, it has been replaced with Iceland moss *(Cetraria islandica)* from the original formula *ga bur 25* (Camphor 25). Irish moss *(Chondrus crispus),* available from Western herbalists, is considered to be very similar to Iceland moss. The suitability of either Iceland moss or Irish moss as a substitute for *rdo dreg* (salted shield) requires further research. Salted shield may also be available from Ayurvedic herbalists as *shaileyam.*

Known Pharmacological Properties

Irish moss has hypolipidemic, antithrombotic, hypotensive, pulmonary demulcent, immunosuppressive, and antidiarrheal actions, reduces gastric secretions, and increases the water content of the gut (Willard 1991).

Herbs That Treat Disorders of the Channels and Blood Vessels

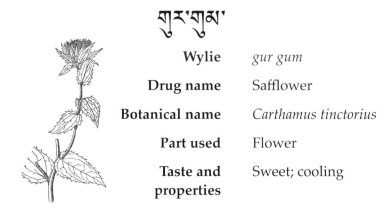

གུར་གུམ་

Wylie	*gur gum*
Drug name	Safflower
Botanical name	*Carthamus tinctorius*
Part used	Flower
Taste and properties	Sweet; cooling

Traditional Actions and Clinical Uses

- Treats all liver disorders: this is one of the Six Excellent Drugs used in many formulas.
- Mends ruptured blood vessels.
- Removes impure blood.
- *kha che gur gum* (saffron) directs the action of a formula to the gallbladder (Dawa 1999).

Procurement and Variants

Safflower (*gur gum*) and the more expensive saffron (*kha che gur gum*) are used interchangeably, although saffron is considered superior. Safflower is available from Chinese herbalists as *hong hua* (红花). Saffron is available at Indian grocery stores and from other sources. Good saffron looks solid red with few or no yellow parts.

Known Pharmacological Properties

- Safflower stimulates the heart muscle at low doses but inhibits it at higher doses. It can increase coronary flow but can constrict other blood vessels. It has hypotensive, anti-inflammatory, analgesic, antipyretic, vasodilatory, hepatoprotective, antimicrobial, uterotonic, bronchoconstrictive, CNS depressant, immunosuppressant, and antithrombotic actions (Chang and But 1986; WHO 2007). Angiogenic action has also been reported.
- Saffron has antiatherosclerotic, antithrombotic, anticancer, sedative, and memory-enhancing actions. It also helps the circulation of blood (WHO 2007).

Additional Reference

Wang, S., Z. Zheng, Y. Weng, Y. Yu, D. Zhang, W. Fan, R. Dai, and Z. Hu. 2004. Angiogenesis and anti-angiogenesis activity of Chinese medicinal herbal extracts. *Life Sciences* 74 (20): 2467–78.

དོམ་མཁྲིས་

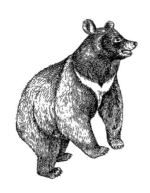

Wylie	*dom mkhris*
Drug name	Bear bile
Latin name	*Ursus sp.*
Part used	Bile
Taste and properties	Bitter and slightly sweet

Traditional Actions and Clinical Uses

- "Constricts the mouth of the channels": bear bile has an important action on the blood system, notably to stop bleeding. It also stops vomiting.
- Controls inflammation associated with fever.
- Stops tissue necrosis and helps grow new healthy tissue: bear bile is often used in the treatment of dark phlegm, especially to help heal damaged lung tissue.

Procurement and Variants

Because of the endangered or near-endangered status of most bear species and the inhumane conditions in which domestic bear bile is harvested, a substitute is advisable. In Chinese medicine, cow gallbladder is known as *niu dan* (牛胆) and is used at a higher dosage in place of bear bile (Bensky and Gamble 1986). Pig gallbladder or *zhu dan* (猪胆) and cow gallstone or *niu huang* (牛黄) may also be considered (Chang and But 1987).

Known Pharmacological Properties

Bear bile has cholagogic, choleretic, gallstone-dissolving, spasmolytic, cardiotonic, hypotensive, antidotal, bacteriostatic, anti-inflammatory, antiallergic, antitussive, expectorant, antiasthmatic, sedative, anticonvulsant, and antipyretic actions (Chang and But 1987).

Herbs That Benefit the Urinary System

གཟེ་མ་

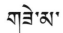

Wylie	*gze ma*
Drug name	Puncture vine
Botanical name	*Tribulus terrestris*
Part used	Fruit
Taste and properties	Sweet; warming

Traditional Actions and Clinical Uses

- Treats cold kidney disorders.
- Treats dysuria.
- Treats lymph *(chu ser)* disorders.
- Treats cold wind disorders: puncture vine is often used in combination with *ba spru* (Himalayan mirabilis), *lca ba* (angelica), *ra mnye* (Solomon's seal), and *nye shing* (asparagus) for the treatment of wind.

Procurement

Puncture vine is available from Western herbalists, from Chinese herbalists as *bai ji li* (白蒺藜), and from Ayurvedic herbalists as *gokshura*.

Known Pharmacological Properties

Puncture vine has antiurolithic, nephroprotective, antimicrobial, cardiotonic, antispasmodic, hepatoprotective, antitumor, diuretic, hypoglycemic, hypotensive, estrogenic, leukopenic, and aphrodisiac actions (Bensky and Gamble 1986; Caldecott 2006; Ross 1999; Williamson 2002).

འཇམ་འབྲས་

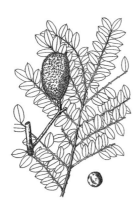

Wylie	*'jam 'bras*
Drug name	Fever nut
Botanical name	*Caesalpinia bonducella* syn. *C. crista*
Part used	Seed
Taste and properties	Acrid; warming

Traditional Actions and Clinical Uses

- Treats cold kidney disorders.
- Because of its acrid taste and warming action, fever nut is also used to treat phlegm disorders.

Procurement

Fever nut may be available from Ayurvedic herbalists as *latakaranja*.

Known Pharmacological Properties

Fever nut has anti-inflammatory, antidiarrheal, antimalarial, antiviral, antiestrogenic, hypoglycemic, hypolipidemic, and uterotonic actions (Williamson 2002).

རྒྱ་ཚྭ་

Wylie	*rgya tshwa*
Drug name	Ammonium chloride
Latin name	*Sal ammoniac*
Taste and properties	Very acrid; sharp

Traditional Actions and Clinical Uses

- Treats urinary retention: along with *gser gyis bye ma* (vermiculite), this is one of the best remedies.
- Treats poisoning.
- Expels parasites.
- Treats channel disorders.
- Removes abnormal growths.
- Ammonium chloride directs the action of a formula to the bladder (Dawa 1999).

Chemical Composition

NH_4Cl

Procurement

Ammonium chloride is available from pharmacy-supply vendors. It may also be available from Chinese herbalists as *lu sha* (卤砂).

ཤུག་པ་ཚེར་ཅན་

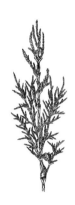

Wylie	*shug pa tsher can*
Drug name	Juniper
Botanical name	*Sabina sp.* syn. *Juniperus sp.*
Part used	Seed and leaf
Taste and properties	Bitter and astringent; cooling

Traditional Actions and Clinical Uses

Reduces fever in the lower part of the body, especially the kidneys.

Procurement and Variants

Many kinds of juniper are used in Tibetan medicine, including *Juniperus formosana, J. tibetica, J. squamata,* and *J. recurva.* Juniper berry is a common Western spice, but juniper leaf is harder to find. It is sometimes sold as incense.

Known Pharmacological Properties

Juniper berry has diuretic, antiviral, antibiotic, and antifungal actions (Willard 1991). Anticancer activity has also been reported.

Additional Reference

Goun, E. A., V. M. Petrichenko, S. U. Solodnikov, T. V. Suhinina, M. A. Kline, G. Cunningham, C. Nguyen, and H. Miles. 2002. Anticancer and antithrombin activity of Russian plants. *Journal of Ethnopharmacology* 81 (3): 337–42.

 བ་སྤྲུ་

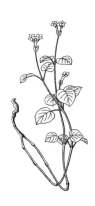

Wylie	*ba spru*
Drug name	Himalayan mirabilis
Botanical name	*Mirabilis himalaica*
Part used	Root
Taste and properties	Sweet and acrid; warming

Traditional Actions and Clinical Uses

- Restores kidney heat and bodily vigor.
- Treats dropsy and accumulation of fluid in the joints.
- Himalayan mirabilis is often used in combination with *lca ba* (angelica), *ra mnye* (Solomon's seal), *gze ma* (puncture vine), and *nye shing* (asparagus) for the treatment of wind.
- Himalayan mirabilis directs the action of a formula to the uterus (Dawa 1999).

སྡིག་སྲིན་

Wylie	*sdig srin*
Drug name	Crab
Part used	Entire animal
Taste and properties	Sweet, slightly acrid; warming, sharp

Traditional Actions and Clinical Uses

Treats urinary retention.

Procurement

Crab is a common foodstuff.

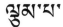

Wylie	*lcam pa*
Drug name	Mallow
Botanical name	*Malva verticillata*
Part used	Seed
Taste and properties	Sweet and astringent; warming

Traditional Actions and Clinical Uses

- Treats dropsy.
- Alleviates thirst.
- Dilates the channels.
- Alleviates diarrhea.
- Alleviates urinary blockage.

Procurement and Variants

Mallow seeds are available from Chinese herbalists as *dong kui zi* (冬葵子). The Chinese drug name subsumes both Chinese mallow *(Malva verticillata)* and Indian mallow *(Abutilon theophrasti)*. The seeds of many varieties of marsh mallow *(Malva sylvestris)*, a close cousin of *Malva verticillata*, are available from gardening stores.

Known Pharmacological Properties

Mallow seed has immunomodulatory and hypoglycemic actions.

References

Gonda, R., M. Tomoda, M. Kanari, N. Shimizu, and H. Yamada. 1990. Constituents of the seed of *Malva verticillata*. VI. Characterization and immunological activities of a novel acidic polysaccharide. *Chemical and Pharmaceutical Bulletin* 38 (10): 2771–4.

Gonda, R., M. Tomoda, N. Shimizu, and M. Kanari. 1990. Characterization of an acidic polysaccharide from the seeds of *Malva verticillata* stimulating the phagocytic activity of cells of the RES. *Planta Medica* 56 (1): 73–6.

Tomoda, M., N. Shimizu, R. Gonda, M. Kanari, H. Yamada, and H. Hikino. 1990. Anti-complementary and hypoglycemic activities of the glycans from the seeds of *Malva verticillata*. *Planta Medica* 56 (2): 168–70.

ཞུ་མཁན་

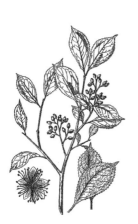

Wylie	*zhu mkhan*
Drug name	Sapphireberry, Asiatic sweetleaf
Botanical name	*Symplocos paniculata*
Part used	Leaf
Taste and properties	Bitter and astringent; neutral

Traditional Actions and Clinical Uses

- Treats fever of the lungs and kidneys.
- Treats spread and disturbed fever.
- Sapphireberry is used in combination with *btsod* (Indian madder), *rgya skyegs* (shellac), and/or *'bri mog* (Tibetan groomwell) to treat fever in the blood and in the lungs and to remove heat from the kidneys.

Procurement and Variants

A closely related species, lodh tree *(Symplocos racemosa)* is available from Ayurvedic herbalists as *lodhra* and is probably a good substitute.

Known Pharmacological Properties

Lodh tree *(Symplocos racemosa)* has antimicrobial, antifibrinolytic, and anti-spasmodic effects (Williamson 2002).

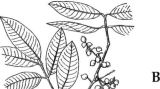

Wylie	*sra 'bras, sa 'bras*
Drug name	Java plum
Botanical name	*Eugenia jambolana* syn. *Syzygium cumini*
Part used	Fruit
Taste and properties	Sweet and sour; warming

Traditional Actions and Clinical Uses

Treats kidney disorders: Java plum is often used in combination with a *'bras* (mango) and *'jam 'bras* (fever nut).

Procurement

Java plum is a common foodstuff in Asia but is hard to find in the West. Extract is sometimes available in liquid or powder form as a food supplement.

Known Pharmacological Properties

Java plum has a well-documented role in the treatment of diabetes mellitus because of its hypoglycemic effects. It can decrease capillary permeability. It also has antibacterial, antipyretic, antidotal, depressant, diuretic, anti-inflammatory, antidiarrheal, and other actions (Williamson 2002).

ཨ་འབྲས་

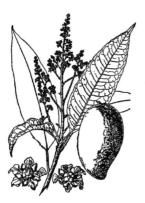

Wylie	*a 'bras*
Drug name	Mango
Botanical name	*Mangifera indica*
Part used	The white substance contained in the kernel
Taste and properties	Sweet, sour, and slightly astringent; warming

Traditional Actions and Clinical Uses

Restores kidney heat.

Procurement

Mango is a common foodstuff.

Known Pharmacological Properties

Mango kernel has anthelmintic, anti-inflammatory, and antimicrobial actions. Most other research pertains to leaf or stem-bark extracts (Ross 1999; Williamson 2002).

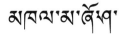

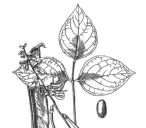

Wylie	*mkhal ma zho sha*
Drug name	Sword bean
Botanical name	*Canavalia gladiata*
Part used	Seeds
Taste and properties	Sweet; oily and neutral

Traditional Actions and Clinical Uses

Lowers kidney fever but restores kidney heat: sword bean can treat both hot and cold kidney disorders.

Procurement

A related species, cowhage *(Mucuna pruriens),* is available from Ayurvedic herbalists as *kapikachu* and has similar effects.

Known Pharmacological Properties

Cowhage has antiparkinson, hypoglycemic, antihemorrhagic, spermatogenic, aphrodisiac, anabolic, analgesic, anti-inflammatory, and antipyretic actions. Indolealkylamines extracted from cowhage have a hallucinogenic action (Ross 1999; Williamson 2002).

གསེར་གྱིས་བྱེ་མ་
གསེར་བྱེ་

Wylie	*gser gyis bye ma, gser bye*
Drug name	Vermiculite
Taste and properties	Salty

Traditional Actions and Clinical Uses

Treats kidney disorders and urinary retention: along with *rgya tshwa* (ammonium chloride), this is one of the best remedies.

Chemical Composition

A typical vermiculite sample contains 38.6% SiO_2, 22.7% MgO, 14.9% Al_2O_3, 9.3% Fe_2O_3, 7.8% K_2O, 1.2% CaO, 0.3% Cr_2O_3, 0.1% Mn_3O_4, and 0.3% Cl (Merck Index 1983).

Procurement

Vermiculite is a common soil additive, available in gardening stores. However, many batches of vermiculite have historically been contaminated with asbestos, a powerful carcinogen. Laboratory tests are available to detect contamination.

Herbs That Benefit the Lungs

ཅུ་གང་

Wylie	*cu gang*
Drug name	Bamboo pith
Botanical name	*Bambusa arundinacea* or *B. textilis*
Part used	Resin
Taste and properties	Bland; cooling

Traditional Actions and Clinical Uses

- Treats all types of hot lung disorders: this is one of the Six Excellent Drugs used in many formulas. It may be taken dissolved in water for lung illnesses (Thubten Phuntsog 2001).
- Treats fever: bamboo pith if often used in combination with *gur gum* (safflower) and other cooling herbs for that purpose.
- Treats fever caused by wounds.

Procurement and Variants

Bamboo pith is available from Ayurvedic herbalists as *lochana*. It is sometimes available from Chinese herbalists as *ju huang jing* (竹黄精), which looks bright white. More often only *tian ju huang* (天竹黄) is available, which is grayish-white, less refined, and probably inferior.

Known Pharmacological Properties

Bamboo pith has an anti-inflammatory action and can reduce the fertility of male rats (Caldecott 2006).

ཤིང་མངར་

Wylie	*shing mngar*
Drug name	Licorice
Botanical name	*Glycyrrhiza glabra* or *G. uralensis*
Part used	Root
Taste and properties	Sweet; neutral

Traditional Actions and Clinical Uses

- Treats lung disorders.
- Treats channel disorders.

Procurement

Licorice is available from Ayurvedic herbalists as *yashtimadhu,* from Chinese herbalists as *gan cao* (甘草), and from Western herbalists.

Known Pharmacological Properties

Licorice has antiulcer, hepatoprotective, antioxidant, antimicrobial, antiviral, anticancer, antiallergic, antipyretic, antispasmodic, antidotal, antitussive, expectorant, hypolipidemic, antidiuretic, antiangiogenic, and anti-inflammatory actions (Chang and But 1986; Williamson 2002).

Additional References

Kobayashi, S., T. Miyamoto, I. Kimura, and M. Kimura. 1995. Inhibitory effect of isoliquiritin, a compound in licorice root, on angiogenesis in vivo and tube formation in vitro. *Biological and Pharmaceutical Bulletin* 18 (10): 1382–6.

Glycyrrhiza glabra monograph. 2005. *Alternative Medicine Review* 10 (3): 230–7.

སྟར་བུ་

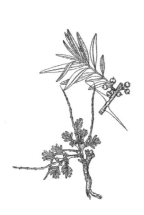

Wylie	*star bu*
Drug name	Sea buckthorn
Botanical name	*Hippophae rhamnoides*
Part used	Fruit
Taste and properties	Sour and astringent; cooling, sharp, light, and coarse

Traditional Actions and Clinical Uses

- Benefits the lungs.
- Promotes the circulation of blood and prevents the formation of phlegm and mucus: sea buckthorn is often used in the treatment of dark phlegm.

Procurement

Sea buckthorn can sometimes be found with Chinese herbalists as *sha ji* (沙棘).

Known Pharmacological Properties

Sea buckthorn has antiarrhythmic and hepatoprotective actions. It can lower cholesterol while increasing HDL-C (Chinese Materia Medica 2002).

Additional Reference

Shukla, S. K., P. Chaudhary, I. P. Kumar, N. Samanta, F. Afrin, M. L. Gupta, U. K. Sharma, A. K. Sinha, Y. K. Sharma, and R. K. Sharma. 2006. Protection from radiation-induced mitochondrial and genomic DNA damage by an extract of *Hippophae rhamnoides*. *Environmental and Molecular Mutagenesis* 47 (9): 647–56.

ক্সুন'འབྲུམ'

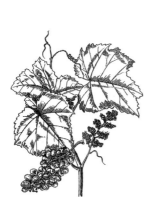

Wylie	*rgun 'brum*
Drug name	Raisin
Botanical name	*Vitis vinifera*
Part used	Fruit
Taste and properties	Sweet and slightly sour; cooling, heavy, and slightly astringent after digestion

Traditional Actions and Clinical Uses

- Treats hot disorders of the lungs.
- Treats fever: raisin is used as a purgative to the treatment of fever and inflammation.

Procurement and Variants

Raisin is a common foodstuff. The very small, yellow, sweet, and seedless grapes from Kashmir are said to be the best (Clark 1995). An organic variety should be used in order to avoid toxicity.

Known Pharmacological Properties

Raisin has antioxidant (Chinese Materia Medica 2002) and antiangiogenic properties. Resveratrol, a component of grape skin, has antioxidant, cardioprotective, anticancer, anti-inflammatory, and neuroprotective actions.

Additional References

Agarwal, C., R. P. Singh, S. Dhanalakshmi, and R. Agarwal. 2004. Anti-angiogenic efficacy of grape seed extract in endothelial cells. *Oncology Reports* 11 (3): 681–5.

Cao, Y., Z. D. Fu, F. Wang, H. Y. Liu, and R. Han. 2005. Anti-angiogenic activity of resveratrol, a natural compound from medicinal plants. *Journal of Asian Natural Products Research* 7 (3): 205–13.

de la Lastra, C. A., and I. Villegas. 2005. Resveratrol as an anti-inflammatory and anti-aging agent: Mechanisms and clinical implications. *Molecular Nutrition and Food Research* 49 (5): 405–30.

Bureau, G., F. Longpré, and M. G. Martinoli. 2008. Resveratrol and quercetin, two natural polyphenols, reduce apoptotic neuronal cell death induced by neuroinflammation. *Journal of Neuroscience Research* 86 (2): 403–10.

King, R. E., J. A. Bomser, and D. B. Min. 2006. Bioactivity of resveratrol. *Comprehensive Reviews in Food Science and Food Safety* 5 (3): 65–70.

Vitaglione, P., S. Sforza, G. Galaverna, C. Ghidini, N. Caporaso, P. P. Vescovi, V. Fogliano, and R. Marchelli. 2005. Bioavailability of trans-resveratrol from red wine in humans. *Molecular Nutrition and Food Research* 49 (5): 495–504.

Wenzel, E., and V. Somoza. 2005. Metabolism and bioavailability of trans-resveratrol. *Molecular Nutrition and Food Research* 49 (5): 472–81.

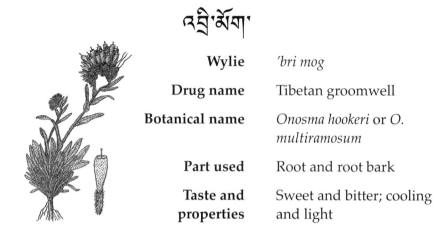

འབྲི་མོག་

Wylie	*'bri mog*
Drug name	Tibetan groomwell
Botanical name	*Onosma hookeri* or *O. multiramosum*
Part used	Root and root bark
Taste and properties	Sweet and bitter; cooling and light

Traditional Actions and Clinical Uses

- Treats fever of the lungs, especially when there is blood in the sputum.
- Alleviates the vomiting of blood.
- Tibetan groomwell is used in combination with *btsod* (Indian madder), *rgya skyegs* (shellac), and/or *zhu mkhan* (sapphireberry) to treat fever in the blood and in the lungs and to remove heat from the kidneys.

Procurement and Variants

Tibetan groomwell is called *zang zi cao* (臟紫草) by Chinese botanists. Chinese groomwell *(Lithospermum erythrorhizon)*, also of the borage family, is used in Chinese medicine with comparable effects and is known as *zi cao* (紫草). Its suitability in the context of Tibetan medicine needs to be verified. In Tibetan medicine, *zhu mkhan* (sapphireberry) is sometimes used as a substitute for Tibetan groomwell.

Known Pharmacological Properties

Chinese groomwell *(Lithospermum erythrorhizon)* has antibiotic, anti-inflammatory, antihistaminic, antiangiogenic, anticancer, and antifertility actions (Bensky and Gamble 1986).

Additional References

Han, K. Y., T. H. Kwon, T. H. Lee, S. J. Lee, S. H. Kim, and J. Kim. 2008. Suppressive effects of *Lithospermum erythrorhizon* extracts on lipopolysaccharide-induced activation of AP-1 and NF-kappaB via mitogen-activated protein kinase pathways in mouse macrophage cells. *BMB Reports* 41 (4): 328–33.

Hisa, T., Y. Kimura, K. Takada, F. Suzuki, and M. Takigawa. 1998. Shikonin, an ingredient of *Lithospermum erythrorhizon*, inhibits angiogenesis in vivo and in vitro. *Anticancer Research* 18 (2A): 783–90.

Kim, E. K., E. Y. Kim, P. D. Moon, J. Y. Um, H. M. Kim, H. S. Lee, Y. Sohn, S. K. Park, H. S. Jung, and N. W. Sohn. 2007. *Lithospermi radix* extract inhibits histamine release and production of inflammatory cytokine in mast cells. *Bioscience, Biotechnology, and Biochemistry* 71 (12): 2886–92.

Xin Chen, Lu Yang, Joost J. Oppenheim, and O. M. Zack Howard. 2002. Cellular pharmacology studies of shikonin derivatives. *Phytotherapy Research* 16 (3): 199–209.

ཨ་ཀྲོང་

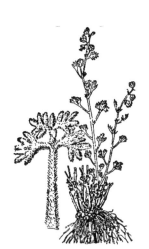

Wylie	*a krong*
Drug name	Sandwort
Botanical name	*Arenaria festucoides* or *Artemisia minor*
Part used	*Arenaria festucoides:* entire plant *Artemisia minor:* stems and leaves
Taste and properties	Sweet and astringent; cooling

Traditional Actions and Clinical Uses

- Treats lung fever.
- Removes pus from the lungs.

Variant

Moxa *(Artemisia argyi* or *A. vulgaris)* may be evaluated for substitution because of its actions on the lungs (Bensky and Gamble 1986; Chang and But 1986). It is available from Chinese herbalists as *ai ye* (艾叶).

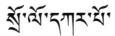

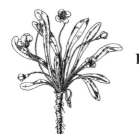

Wylie	*sro lo dkar po*
Botanical name	*Pegaeophyton scapiflorum* syn. *Cochlearia scapiflorum*
Part used	Entire plant
Taste and properties	Sweet; cooling

Traditional Actions and Clinical Uses

* Treats hot lung disorders and other lung disorders.
* Treats turbid fever and infectious fever.

Procurement and Variants

The red variant, *sro lo dmar po (Rhodiola sp.)*, is sometimes available from Chinese herbalists as *hong jing tian* (红景天).

Known Pharmacological Properties

The red variant, *sro lo dmar po (Rhodiola sp.)* has antioxidant, endurance-enhancing, and sedative actions (Chinese Materia Medica 2002). A cardiopulmonary protective action has also been reported.

Additional Reference

Rhodiola rosea monograph. 2002. *Alternative Medicine Review* 7 (5): 421–3.

Panaceas

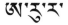

Wylie	*a ru ra*
Drug name	Chebulic myrobalan
Botanical name	*Terminalia chebula*
Part used	Fruit without seed
Taste and properties	Astringent, sweet, and slightly sour; neutral

Traditional Actions and Clinical Uses

- Detoxifies, balances the three humors, and treats all diseases whether hot or cold: this is the drug most employed in Tibetan medicine. It is employed in most herbal formulations, evidently to support the patient's bodily constituents (Dawa 1999). It is attributed quasi-miraculous healing properties and heavenly origins. The Medicine Buddha is represented holding a fresh chebulic myrobalan plant in his right hand and a begging bowl containing dried chebulic myrobalan fruits in his left hand. Several types of chebulic myrobalan are described in traditional texts, including *a ru rnam rgyal* (victorious myrobalan), said to grow in heaven.
- Lowers fever of the blood.
- Treats infections.

Procurement

Chebulic myrobalan is available from Ayurvedic herbalists as *haritaki* and from Chinese herbalists as *he zi* (诃子). It is also sometimes available in Indian grocery stores as *harde*.

Known Pharmacological Properties

Chebulic myrobalan has cardiotonic, antianaphylactic, antitumor, antibacterial, antifungal, antiviral, hepatoprotective, hypolipidemic, antiulcer, and other actions (Caldecott 2006; Williamson 2002).

Remark

The pit of chebulic myrobalan is considered toxic and should not be used.

Additional Reference

Saleem, A., M. Husheem, P. Härkönen, and K. Pihlaja. 2002. Inhibition of cancer cell growth by crude extract and the phenolics of *Terminalia chebula* Retz. fruit. *Journal of Ethnopharmacology* 81 (3): 327–36.

བ་རུ་ར་

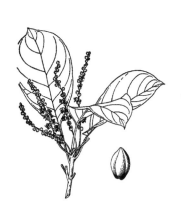

Wylie	*ba ru ra*
Drug name	Beleric myrobalan
Botanical name	*Terminalia belerica* syn. *Myrobalanus bellirica*
Part used	Fruit
Taste and properties	Astringent and slightly sour; neutral

Traditional Actions and Clinical Uses

Treats wind disorders, lymph *(chu ser)* disorders, and combined bile and phlegm disorders: beleric myrobalan is most often used in combination with *a ru ra* (chebulic myrobalan) and *skyu ru ra* (amla).

Procurement

Beleric myrobalan is available from Ayurvedic herbalists as *bibhitaki*.

Known Pharmacological Properties

Beleric myrobalan has antioxidant, antiasthmatic, expectorant, antitussive, hypotensive, hypolipidemic, hepatoprotective, antiulcer, and other actions (Caldecott 2006; Williamson 2002).

Remark

The pit of beleric myrobalan is considered toxic and should not be used.

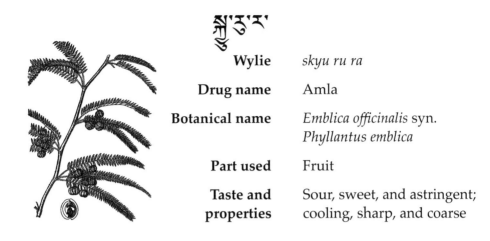

 སྐྱུ་རུ་ར་

Wylie	*skyu ru ra*
Drug name	Amla
Botanical name	*Emblica officinalis* syn. *Phyllantus emblica*
Part used	Fruit
Taste and properties	Sour, sweet, and astringent; cooling, sharp, and coarse

Traditional Actions and Clinical Uses

- Treats combined bile and phlegm disorders.
- Cleanses impure blood.
- Treats recent liver ailments.
- Amla is most often used in combination with *a ru ra* (chebulic myrobalan) and *ba ru ra* (beleric myrobalan).

Procurement

Amla is available from Ayurvedic herbalists as *amalaki*. It is also sometimes available in Indian grocery stores.

Known Pharmacological Properties

Amla has hypolipidemic, antiviral, antidotal, hepatoprotective, hypoglycemic, immunomodulatory, antioxidant, antimicrobial, anti-inflammatory, and antipyretic actions (Williamson 2002).

Remark

The pit of amla is considered toxic and should not be used.

བྲག་ཞུན་

Wylie	*brag zhun*
Drug name	Mineral pitch
Latin name	*Asphaltum*
Part used	Processed exudate
Taste and properties	Bitter and sweet; cooling

Traditional Actions and Clinical Uses

- Mineral pitch is one of the most important remedies for liver disorders.
- Treats all types of fever, especially of the stomach, liver, and kidneys.
- Treats wind disorders.
- Treats multiple-humor disorders.
- Rejuvenates: mineral pitch is used in essence extraction.

Procurement

Mineral pitch is often sold in capsules by Ayurvedic vendors as *shilajit* or *shilajatu*, but the quality is unpredictable. It is not used in its native form but purified by water extraction.

Known Pharmacological Properties

Mineral pitch has nootropic, anxiolytic, hypolipidemic, hypoglycemic, antiulcer, and anti-inflammatory actions. It has been found helpful in opiate withdrawal in mice (Caldecott 2006).

Additional References

Agarwal, S. P., R. Khanna, R. Karmarkar, M. K. Anwer, and R. K. Khar. 2007. *Shilajit*: A review. *Phytotherapy Research* 21 (5): 401–5.

Ghosal, S., J. P. Reddy, and V. K. Lal. 1976. *Shilajit* I: Chemical constituents. *Journal of Pharmaceutical Sciences* 65 (5): 772–3.

Park, J. S., G. Y. Kim, and K. Han. 2006. The spermatogenic and ovogenic effects of chronically administered *Shilajit* to rats. *Journal of Ethnopharmacology* 107 (3): 349–53.

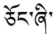

Wylie	*cong zhi*
Drug name	Calcite
Latin name	*Calcitum*
Taste and properties	Warming

Traditional Actions and Clinical Uses

- Treats hot phlegm: calcite is often used in the treatment of phlegm and dark phlegm. For this purpose it may also be used singly after purification by fire and ground with milk (Thubten Phuntsog 2001).
- Rejuvenates: calcite is used in essence extraction.
- Stops diarrhea.

Chemical Composition

Calcium carbonate, $CaCO_3$

Procurement

Calcite is available from Chinese herbalists as *han shui shi* (寒水石).

Remark

Calcite must be detoxified prior to use. This is done by breaking it into small pieces and boiling it in water for twenty minutes. Foam and other impurities should be removed. The calcite is then washed in water eight or nine times, and finally ground into a flat mortar while adding milk.

ར་མཉེ་

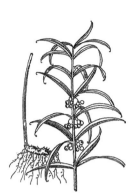

Wylie	*ra mnye*
Drug name	Solomon's seal
Botanical name	*Polygonatum cirrhifolium*
Part used	Root
Taste and properties	Sweet, bitter, and astringent; warming

Traditional Actions and Clinical Uses

- Increases the life span.
- Treats accumulation of lymph *(chu ser)* in the joints.
- Restores digestive heat and strengthens the spleen.
- Strengthens the bones, tendons, and ligaments.
- Treats wind disorders: Solomon's seal is most often used in combination with *lca ba* (angelica), *nye shing* (asparagus), *gze ma* (puncture vine), and *ba spru* (Himalayan mirabilis) for the general treatment of wind disorders.

Procurement and Variants

Solomon's seal is available from Chinese herbalists as *huang jing* (黄精). Under that Chinese drug name are included many possible varieties of *Polygonatum*, including *P. cirrhifolium, P. sibiricum, P. cyrtomena, P. macropodium,* and *P. kingianum.*

Known Pharmacological Properties

Solomon's seal has hypotensive, hypolipidemic, antimicrobial, and hypoglycemic actions. One should note that Solomon's seal's hypoglycemic action is preceded by a temporary hyperglycemic effect due to the herb's carbohydrate contents (Chang and But 1987).

ཉེ་ཤིང་

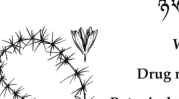

Wylie	*nye shing*
Drug name	Asparagus
Botanical name	*Asparagus cochinchinensis* or *A. racemosus*
Part used	Root
Taste and properties	Bitter, astringent, and sweet; warming

Traditional Actions and Clinical Uses

- Restores physical vigor and kidney heat and treats cold disorders: asparagus is most often used in combination with *lca ba* (angelica), *ra mnye* (Solomon's seal), *gze ma* (puncture vine), and *ba spru* (Himalayan mirabilis) for the general treatment of wind disorders.
- Relieves itching.
- Treats chronic hidden fever.

Procurement and Variants

Medicinal asparagus is available from Ayurvedic herbalists as *shatavari* and from Chinese herbalists as *tian men dong* (天门冬).

Known Pharmacological Properties

Medicinal asparagus has anticancer, adaptogenic, antibiotic, antitussive, bronchodilatory, hepatoprotective, antiulcer, galactagogue, antioxidant, and immunomodulatory actions (Caldecott 2006; Williamson 2002).

Less Commonly Used Herbs

The following herbs are less frequently employed and were not described in the first part of this chapter. Significant problems of identification persist. The table below summarizes some of the information—often not corroborated—that could be obtained, sorted by Tibetan name:

Tibetan Name	Possible Latin Names	English Name or Description
ka bed	*Cucurbita sp.*	Squash seed
ko byi la	*Strychnos nux-vomica*	Nux vomica
skra bzang zil pa	*Corydalis impatiens*	
kham bu	*Prunus armeniaca*	Apricot kernel
khrag khrog pa	*Lepidium apetalum*	
khre ma		Millet
khron bu	*Euphorbia stracheyi*	
gangs thigs		Smithsonite
go thal	*Carum carvi*	Calcined caraway
go bye	*Semecarpus anacardium*	Marking nut
go yu	*Areca catechu*	Betel nut
gres ma	*Iris sp.*	Iris
'gron thal	*Cypraea sp.*	Calcined cowrie shell
rgya ru	*Capricornis sumatraensis*	Mainland serow horn
sgong thog pa	*Erysimum sp.*	Wallflower
sgro puShpa		A red flower
sgron shing	*Pinus sp.*	Pine node
sngon bu	*Cyananthus lobatus*	Trailing bellflower
lcags	*Ferrum*	Iron
lce tsha	*Ranunculus sp.*	Buttercup

Tibetan Name	Possible Latin Names	English Name or Description
lce myang tshwa		A white natural salt with a red hue found in water
nya phyis		Mother-of-pearl
snya lo	*Polygonum sp.*	
tang kun nag po	*Selinum wallichianum*	Wallich milk parsley
rta lpags	*Lamiophlomis rotata*	
stong ri zil pa	*Corydalis sp.*	Fumewort
tha ram	*Plantago sp.*	Plantago
thang phrom	*Anisodus tanguticus, Datura stramonium, Hyoscyamus niger, Mandragora chinghaiensis, Nicandra physaloides, Przewalskia tangutica*, etc.	Nightshade
thar nu	*Euphorbia wallichii*	Wallich spurge
da byid smug po	*Batrachuperus sp.*	Stream salamander
dan khra	*Croton tiglium*	Purging croton
dan rog	*Ricinus communis*	Castor oil plant
dung thal	*Strombus sp.*	Calcined conch shell
mda' rgyus	*Abrus precatorius*	Precatory bean
mdung rtsi		Goethite
ldong ros		Realgar
nim pa	*Azadirachta indica*, syn. *Melia azadirachta*	Neem tree
pa yag rtsa ba	*Lancea tibetica*	Tibetan lancea
pu Shkara mU la	*Inula racemosa*	Pushkarmool
spyang tsher	*Morina sp., Carduus sp., Cirsium sp.*	Thistle
spra ba	*Leontopodium sp.*	

Tibetan Name	Possible Latin Names	English Name or Description
phur thal	*Artemisia sp.*	Calcined Artemisia
bya rkang	*Delphinium caeruleum*	Larkspur
bya rgod spos	*Delphinium brunonianum*	Larkspur
byi rug	*Elsholtzia densa, E. eriostachya*	
dbang po lag pa	*Orchis sp.*	Salep orchid
'bras yos	*Oryza sativa*	Parched rice
'bri rta sa 'dzin	*Fragaria nubicola, F. orientalis*	Wild strawberry
'brong khrag	*Bos grunniens*	Wild yak blood
ming can nag po	*Pulicaria insignis*	
mu tig		Pearl
mu zi		Sulfur
mon cha ra	*Quercus semecarpifolia*	Himalayan oak acorn
myang rtsi spras	*Coptis sp.*	Goldthread
sman lcags	*Magnetitum*	Magnetite
rtsab ru tshwa		Crag halite
tshar bong	*Artemisia sp.*	Artemisia
tshur nag	*Fibroferitum*	Black alunite
mtsho tshwa		Lake salt
mdze tshwa		Glauber's salt
'dzin pa	*Aconitum sp.*	Blue aconite
wa yi glo ba	*Vulpes sp.*	Lung of fox or other large animal
rwa tshwa		Salt made from horn
'om bu	*Myricaria sp.*	German tamarisk
ya bakSha ra		Saltpeter
yu gu shing nag po	*Sambucus sp.*	Elderberry
g.ya' kyi ma	*Chrysosplenium sp.*	Golden saxifrage

Tibetan Name	Possible Latin Names	English Name or Description
g.yer ma	Zanthoxylum sp.	Sichuan pepper
ra sug	Silene sp.	Campion
ri sho	Ligularia sp.	Leopard plant
srad dkar	Oxytropis sp.	Locoweed
la la phud	Aegopodium podagraria, Foeniculum vulgare, or Cnidium monnieri	Bishop's weed, fennel, or Monnier's snowparsley
lug mur	Phlomis younghusbandii	
klu bdud rdo rje	Codonopsis nervosa	Bonnet bellflower
sha ru	Cervus sp.	Deer horn
se rgod bar shun	Rosa sp.	Middle bark of Rosa sp.
so cha	Sesbania grandiflora	Hummingbird tree
gser gyi phud bu	Luffa aegyptiaca	Sponge gourd

Principles of Herb Compounding

Choice of Herbs

Traditionally, in compounding herbs one needs to consider their taste, postdigestive taste, and inherent healing properties as described in detail in Chapters 19 and 20 of the Explanatory (Second) Tantra. In summary, sweet, sour, salty, and pungent tastes benefit wind disorders. Bitter, sweet, and astringent tastes treat bile. Pungent, sour, and salty tastes treat phlegm. Certain herbs direct a formula to a specific site or organ in particular (Dawa 1999):

- *dzA ti* (nutmeg) for the heart
- *cu gang* (bamboo pith) for the lungs
- *gur gum* (safflower) for the liver
- *sug smel* (green cardamom) for the kidneys
- *li shi* (clove) for the channels and blood vessels
- *se 'bru* (pomegranate) for the stomach
- *kha che gur gum* (saffron) for the gallbladder
- *dug mo nyung* (kurchi) for the small intestine
- *ru rta* (costus) for the large intestine
- *ba spru* (Himalayan mirabilis) for the uterus
- *rgya tshwa* (ammonium chloride) for the bladder
- *mdung rtsi* (goethite) for the eyes
- *ba sha ka* (Malabar nut tree) for the blood

In addition, herbs are combined to counteract each other's side effects. In general, herb formulas tax the digestive system, therefore *se 'bru* (pomegranate), *pi pi ling* (long pepper), and similar herbs are often added to formulas to support the digestive system. It must also be remembered that treating a given humor entails balancing the other two humors in equal measure.

Formula Composition

The composition of formulas is sometimes explained hierarchically with the analogy of a king, embodied by the herb or group of herbs that perform the main therapeutic action. This is followed by the queen or ministers that perform complementary functions, then subjects that assist the main action and counterbalance any undesired effect, and finally the horse or vehicle that aids in assimilation. The vehicle is often one of the following:

- For wind disorders, *bu ram* (raw cane sugar)
- For blood and bile disorders, *ka ra* (white rock sugar)
- For phlegm and lymph *(chu ser)* disorders, *sbrang rtsi* (honey)
- The boiled rind of *se 'bru* (pomegranate) is also often used as a binding agent to form pills from powdered material.

Examples of formulas described hierarchically can be found in the treatment of dark phlegm using stone recipes, in the formula *bsam 'phel nor bu* (Wish-fulfilling Jewel), and elsewhere (Dawa 1999).

The more common way herbs are combined into a formula is by combining several smaller formulas or building-block combinations (see below) together or with additional herbs. It should be noted that in modern practice the physician does not formulate the herb combination but relies on standard formulas, as described in the next chapter.

Building-Block Herb Combinations

The rest of this chapter describes often-used synergistic herb combinations. These form groups that work well together and form the basis of many formulas.

The Excellent Drug Combinations

Six Excellent Drugs (bzang po drug)

- *cu gang* (bamboo pith)
- *gur gum* (safflower)
- *li shi* (clove)
- *sug smel* (green cardamom)
- *dzA ti* (nutmeg)
- *ka ko la* (black cardamom)

Four Excellent Drugs (bzang po bzhi) or Four Warming Drugs (drod bzhi)

- *li shi* (clove)
- *sug smel* (green cardamom)
- *dzA ti* (nutmeg)
- *ka ko la* (black cardamom)

Three Excellent Drugs (bzang po gsum) or Three Warming Drugs (drod gsum)

- *sug smel* (green cardamom)
- *dzA ti* (nutmeg)
- *ka ko la* (black cardamom)

Four Cooling Drugs (bsil bzhi)

- *cu gang* (bamboo pith)
- *gur gum* (safflower)
- *li shi* (clove)
- *sug smel* (green cardamom)

Three Cooling Drugs (bsil gsum)

- *cu gang* (bamboo pith)
- *gur gum* (safflower)
- *li shi* (clove)

The five related combinations are summarized in the table below:

Combination	Herb	Herb function	Combination	
Six Excellent Drugs	Four Warming Drugs or Four Excellent Drugs	*cu gang* (bamboo pith)	Benefits the lungs, treats bile	Three Cooling Drugs	Four Cooling Drugs
		gur gum (safflower)	Benefits the liver, treats bile		
		li shi (clove)	Benefits the life channel, treats wind		
		sug smel (green cardamom)	Benefits the kidneys, treats phlegm	Three Warming Drugs or Three Excellent Drugs	
		dzA ti (nutmeg)	Benefits the heart, treats wind		
		ka ko la (black cardamom)	Benefits the spleen, treats phlegm		

Actions

The Six Excellent Drug combination is a very balanced, all-around beneficial combination that can treat a variety of disorders. It addresses the five major internal organs (lungs, liver, kidneys, heart, and spleen). It contains two herbs to treat each of the three humors. It has the same number of cool and warm herbs and thus can be used for both hot and cold conditions.

Variations on the above can be made cooling or warming depending on the herbs omitted. The Three Warming Drugs and the Four Warming Drugs include *sug smel* (green cardamom), a cooling herb, for balance. Likewise the Three Cooling Drugs and the Four Cooling Drugs include *li shi* (clove), a warming herb, for balance.

The Pungent Drug Combinations

Three Pungent Drugs (tsha ba gsum)

- *pi pi ling* (long pepper)
- *na le sham* (black pepper)
- *sman sga* (ginger)

Five Pungent Drugs (tsha ba lnga)

- *pi pi ling* (long pepper)
- *na le sham* (black pepper)
- *sman sga* (ginger)
- *tsi tra ka* (wild leadwort)
- *dbyi mong* (clematis)

Actions

- The Three Pungent Drugs treat cold phlegm and improve the appetite.
- The Five Pungent Drugs treat cold phlegm, improve the appetite, and increase the digestive heat.

The Three Fruits (*'bras bu gsum*)

Composition

- *a ru ra* (chebulic myrobalan) balances the three humors and is auspicious and wish-fulfilling.
- *ba ru ra* (beleric myrobalan) treats phlegm, bile, and lymph (*chu ser*) disorders.
- *skyu ru ra* (amla) treats phlegm, blood, and bile disorders.

Actions

- Treats fever.
- Separates pure blood from diseased blood: this decoction is often used to gather scattered fever.
- Balances wind that affects the blood.
- Helps ripen fever.
- Treats chronic fever and fatigue.

The Three Salts *(tshwa sna gsum)*

Composition

- *rgya tshwa* (ammonium chloride)
- *rgyam tshwa* (rock salt)
- *kha ru tshwa* (black salt)

Actions

The Three Salts treat wind and phlegm and improve digestion.

The Five Roots *(rtsa ba lnga)*

Composition

- *lca ba* (angelica)
- *ba spru* (Himalayan mirabilis)
- *ra mnye* (Solomon's seal)
- *gze ma* (puncture vine)
- *nye shing* (asparagus)

Actions

The Five Roots are a rejuvenating combination used in the treatment of wind. This combination increases digestion, physical vigor, and kidney heat. It is very suitable for elderly and debilitated patients or whenever the bodily constituents are depleted.

The Three Seeds *('bras sna gsum)*

Composition

- a *'bras* (mango)
- sra *'bras* (Java plum)
- *'jam 'bras* (fever nut)

Actions

The Three Seeds warm the kidneys.

Lymph Three *(chu ser sman gsum)*

Composition

- *spos dkar* (frankincense)
- *thal ka rdo rje* (foetid cassia)
- *so ma rA dza* (aibika)

Actions

Lymph Three treats lymph *(chu ser)* disorders. Note that this herb combination is hard to digest.

The Three Bitters *(tig ta gsum)*

Composition

- *rgya tig* (Indian chiretta)
- *bod tig* (Tibetan chiretta)
- *bal tig* (Nepalese chiretta)

Actions

The Three Bitters lower fever associated with bile and blood disorders and treat fever of the liver and gallbladder. This combination can be used whenever *tig ta* (chiretta) is called for if the three herbs are available. Most often *rgya tig* (Indian chiretta) is used alone.

The Three Reds and the Four Reds

Three Reds (dmar gsum)

- *btsod* (Indian madder)
- *rgya skyegs* (shellac)
- *'bri mog* (Tibetan groomwell) or *zhu mkhan* (sapphireberry)

Four Reds (dmar bzhi)

- *btsod* (Indian madder)
- *rgya skyegs* (shellac)
- *'bri mog* (Tibetan groomwell)
- *zhu mkhan* (sapphireberry)

Actions

The Three Reds and Four Reds treat fever in the blood and in the lungs and remove heat from the kidneys.

The Two Sandalwoods and the Three Precious Woods

Two Sandalwoods (tsan dan gnyis)

- *tsan dan dkar po* (sandalwood)
- *tsan dan dmar po* (red sandalwood)

Three Precious Woods (shing mchog gsum)

- *tsan dan dkar po* (sandalwood)
- *tsan dan dmar po* (red sandalwood)
- *a ga ru* (eaglewood)

Actions

- The Two Sandalwoods treat moderate fevers.
- The Three Precious Woods also treat moderate fevers but are more focused on wind and on the heart.

The Three Eaglewoods (a gar rigs gsum)

Composition

- *a ga ru* (eaglewood)
- *ar skya* (Chinese eaglewood)
- *ar dmar* (red eaglewood)

Actions

The action of the Three Eaglewoods is similar to that of *a ga ru* (eaglewood).

Indra Four (indra bzhi)

Composition

- *dug mo nyung* (kurchi)
- *bong nga dkar po* (white aconite)
- *li ga dur* (cranesbill)
- *ba le ka* (birthwort)

Actions

This is a cooling combination that affects the internal organs. When added to *ga bur 25* (Camphor 25), it further relieves fever and inflammation of the hollow organs.

Balancing Four *(cha mnyam bzhi)*

Composition

- *rgyam tshwa* (rock salt)
- *bca' sga* (fresh ginger)
- *a ru ra* (chebulic myrobalan)
- *pi pi ling* (long pepper)

Actions

This combination is a foundation formula for the treatment of cold phlegm.

The Two Myrrhs *(gu gul gnyis)*

Composition

- *gu gul* (myrrh)
- *spos dkar* (frankincense)

Actions

The Two Myrrhs in combination treat lymph *(chu ser)* disorders.

The Two Cumins *(zi ra gnyis)*

Composition

- *zi ra dkar po* (cumin)
- *zi ra nag po* (fennelflower)

Actions

The Two Cumins benefit the stomach, improve the appetite and increase digestive heat.

Elecampane Four *(ma nu bzhi)*

Composition

* *ma nu pa tra* (elecampane)
* *kaNDa ka ri* (two-flowered raspberry)
* *sle tres* (moonseed)
* *sga skya* (galangal)

Actions

Elecampane Four is used to treat recently acquired fever, to gather or ripen contagious fever, or to make hidden fever manifest. It also treats phlegm, dark phlegm, pain caused by blood disorders, and void fever.

Pomegranate Combinations

Pomegranate Four (se 'bru bzhi pa)

* *se 'bru* (pomegranate)
* *shing tsha* (cinnamon)
* *sug smel* (green cardamom)
* *pi pi ling* (long pepper)

Variation 1, Pomegranate Four

* *se 'bru* (pomegranate)
* *shing tsha* (cinnamon)
* *sug smel* (green cardamom)
* *sman sga* (ginger), *sga skya* (galangal), or *dong gra* (lesser galangal)

Variation 2, Pomegranate Four

* *se 'bru* (pomegranate)
* *sug smel* (green cardamom)
* *gur gum* (safflower)
* *pi pi ling* (long pepper)

Variation 3, Pomegranate Four

* *se 'bru* (pomegranate)
* *shing tsha* (cinnamon)
* *gur gum* (safflower)
* *sman sga* (ginger), *sga skya* (galangal), or *dong gra* (lesser galangal)

Pomegranate Five (se 'bru lnga pa)

- *se 'bru* (pomegranate)
- *shing tsha* (cinnamon)
- *sug smel* (green cardamom)
- *pi pi ling* (long pepper)
- *sman sga* (ginger), *sga skya* (galangal), or *dong gra* (lesser galangal)

Pomegranate Sanctuary (se 'bru dwangs ma gnas 'jog)

- *se 'bru* (pomegranate)
- *shing tsha* (cinnamon)
- *sug smel* (green cardamom)
- *pi pi ling* (long pepper)
- *gur gum* (safflower)

Actions

The pomegranate combinations all increase digestive heat with variations that depend on the exact herb combination. Adding *gur gum* (safflower) aids the liver in transforming the chyme into blood, thereby improving assimilation of food and drink.

Commonly Used Herbal Formulas

Formulas That Treat Wind Disorders

bi ma la'i sbyor ba

Vimalamitra's Formula

dzA ti (nutmeg)	Treat heart wind
a ru ra (chebulic myrobalan)	
spos dkar (frankincense)	
a ga ru (eaglewood)	
gi waM (elephant or ox gallstone)	Empirical anticonvulsant and hypotensive
shing kun (asafetida)	Treats heart wind
cu gang (bamboo pith)	With *dzA ti* (nutmeg) above, form the Six Excellent Drugs, which balance the three humors and benefit the six internal organs
ka ko la (black cardamom)	
sug smel (green cardamom)	
li shi (clove)	
gur gum (safflower)	
go snyod (caraway)	Treats heart wind and fever
tsan dan dkar po (white sandalwood)	Two Sandalwoods; treat fever
tsan dan dmar po (red sandalwood)	
ba ru ra (beleric myrobalan)	Three Fruits (with the above); balance the three humors
skyu ru ra (amla)	
seng ldeng (catechu tree)	Treat heart wind
snying zho sha (lapsi tree)	
sgog thal (calcined garlic)	
li ga dur (cranesbill)	Cools fever and detoxifies

Treats wind in the heart.

sems kyi bde skyid

Mental Happiness

shing kun (asafetida)	Treat heart wind
bong nga nag po (dark-blue aconite)	
sga skya (galangal)	Three Pungent Drugs; treat cold phlegm and improve the appetite
na le sham (black pepper)	
pi pi ling (long pepper)	
'brong khrag (wild yak blood)	Treat heart wind
kha ru tshwa (black salt)	
snying zho sha (lapsi tree)	
ru rta (costus)	
dzA ti (nutmeg)	
li shi (clove)	
a ga ru (eaglewood)	
go yu (betel nut)	Benefits the kidneys
ri bong snying (hare heart)	Treats heart wind

- Treats wind disorders of the life channel.
- Treats all types of wind disorders.

srog 'dzin 11

Life-sustaining Wind 11

a ga ru (eaglewood)	Treat wind in the heart and in the life channel
dzA ti (nutmeg)	
snying zho sha (lapsi tree)	
cu gang (bamboo pith)	Rejuvenates
spos dkar (frankincense)	Dries up lymph *(chu ser)* and benefits the heart indirectly
ru rta (costus)	Treats disorders of the life-sustaining wind

a ru ra (chebulic myrobalan)	Balances the humors
nA ga ge sar (silk cotton tree)	Benefits the heart
li shi (clove)	Treat wind in the heart and in the life channel
ri bong snying (hare heart)	
shing kun (asafetida)	

- Treats wind disorders that affect the heart and life channels.
- Treats mental disorders.
- Treats pain in the upper part of the body, especially the upper back, chest, breasts, and liver.

a gar 8

Eaglewood 8

a ga ru (eaglewood)	Treat heart wind and fever
dzA ti (nutmeg)	
snying zho sha (lapsi tree)	
cu gang (bamboo pith)	Treats fever
spos dkar (frankincense)	Dries up lymph (*chu ser*) and benefits the heart indirectly
ru rta (costus)	Treats wind and supports the digestive heat
a ru ra (chebulic myrobalan)	Supports the three humors, treats fever
nA ga ge sar (silk cotton tree)	Treats fever

- Treats wind that affects the heart.
- Benefits the heart in cases of spread fever or disturbed fever.

a gar 15

Eaglewood 15

a ga ru (eaglewood)	
snying zho sha (lapsi tree)	
tsan dan dkar po (white sandalwood)	
tsan dan dmar po (red sandalwood)	Similar to Eaglewood 8 but less focused on the heart
dzA ti (nutmeg)	
cu gang (bamboo pith)	
gur gum (safflower)	
sro lo dkar po (*Pegaeophyton scapiflorum*)	
a ru ra (chebulic myrobalan)	
ba ru ra (beleric myrobalan)	
skyu ru ra (amla)	
ma nu pa tra (elecampane)	Decoction of Seven Precious Ingredients
sle tres (moonseed)	
kaNDa ka ri (two-flowered raspberry)	
sga skya (galangal)	

- Relieves pain all over the body caused by wind affecting the blood.
- Alleviates cough with frothy mucus that occurs in the morning.

a gar 20

Eaglewood 20

a ga ru (eaglewood)	Eaglewood 8
dzA ti (nutmeg)	
snying zho sha (lapsi tree)	
cu gang (bamboo pith)	
spos dkar (frankincense)	
ru rta (costus)	
a ru ra (chebulic myrobalan)	
nA ga ge sar (silk cotton tree)	
tsan dan dmar po (red sandalwood)	Treats blood, wind, and fever
gi waM (elephant or ox gallstone)	Treats fever
li shi (clove)	Treats wind and fever
bse yab (Chinese quince)	Treats bile
gur gum (safflower)	Cools the blood, mends the blood vessels
ma nu pa tra (elecampane)	Treats blood, wind, and recent fever
bse ru'i rwa (rhinoceros horn)	Treat toxic fever
nya phyis (mother-of-pearl)	
ko byi la (nux vomica)	
ri bong snying (hare heart)	Treats wind
'bri rta sa 'dzin (wild strawberry)	Treats inflammation of the channels
skyu ru ra (amla)	Cleanses impure blood

- Treats wind that affects the blood.
- Treats fever or inflammation associated with wind.
- Effective for paralysis, numbness of the extremities, Parkinsonism, stroke, and hypertension.

a gar 35

Eaglewood 35

a ga ru (eaglewood)	Three Eaglewoods; treat fever of the heart and life channel and pacify wind
ar skya (Chinese eaglewood)	
ar dmar (red eaglewood)	
tsan dan dkar po (white sandalwood)	Two Sandalwoods; treat fever
tsan dan dmar po (red sandalwood)	
dzA ti (nutmeg)	Six Excellent Drugs; balance the three humors and benefit the six internal organs
li shi (clove)	
cu gang (bamboo pith)	
gur gum (safflower)	
sug smel (green cardamom)	
ka ko la (black cardamom)	
a ru ra (chebulic myrobalan)	Decoction of Seven Precious Ingredients
ba ru ra (beleric myrobalan)	
skyu ru ra (amla)	
sle tres (moonseed)	
sga skya (galangal)	
kaNDa ka ri (two-flowered raspberry)	
ma nu pa tra (elecampane)	
ba sha ka (Malabar nut tree)	Cool the blood
tig ta (chiretta)	
hong len (picrorhiza grass)	
spos dkar (frankincense)	Two Myrrhs; treat lymph *(chu ser)* disorders and thus benefit the heart indirectly
gu gul (myrrh)	

gla rtsi (musk)	Remove fever
ko byi la (nux vomica)	
nA ga ge sar (silk cotton tree)	
ru rta (costus)	
a byag gzer 'joms (Tartar chrysanthemum)	Alleviate pain
ming can nag po (Pulicaria insignis)	
sha chen (wild yak heart)	
bong nga nag po (dark-blue aconite)	
tsher sngon (blue poppy)	
snying zho sha (lapsi tree)	Treats wind in the heart and fever
se 'bru (pomegranate)	Supports the digestive system
sro lo dkar po (Pegaeophyton scapiflorum)	Removes lung fever

- Treats wind disorders associated with fever or inflammation.
- Eases breathing.
- Alleviates nonlocal pain and pain in the upper back caused by an excess of wind in the blood.

Formulas That Treat Bile Disorders

skyu ru 25

Amla 25

skyu ru ra (amla)	Cool the blood
ba sha ka (Malabar nut tree)	
ba le ka (birthwort)	
pri yang ku (nodding dragonhead)	Treat and prevent dark phlegm
'u su (coriander)	
hong len (picrorhiza grass)	
brag zhun (mineral pitch)	Cool the liver
ut pal (Himalayan poppy)	
spang rtsi do bo (Pterocephalus hookeri)	
gur gum (safflower)	
gi waM (elephant or ox gallstone)	Cool down fever
tsan dan dmar po (red sandalwood)	
btsod (Indian madder)	Three Reds; treat fever in the blood
rgya skyegs (shellac)	
'bri mog (groomwell)	
pu shel rtse (noble dendrobium)	Cool the blood, detoxify, support the digestive system, and balance the humors
li ga dur (cranesbill)	
tig ta (chiretta)	
a ru ra (chebulic myrobalan)	
ba ru ra (beleric myrobalan)	
gser gyi me tog (bolenggua)	
ru rta (costus)	

ma nu pa tra (elecampane)	Variation of Elecampane Four; treat recently acquired fever
kaNDa ka ri (two-flowered raspberry)	
sle tres (moonseed)	
star bu (sea buckthorn)	Promotes the circulation of blood

- Treats blood disorders.
- Lowers blood pressure.
- Harmonizes the flow of menses.

gi waM 9

Gallstone 9

gi waM (elephant or ox gallstone)	Treat fever of the liver
gur gum (safflower)	
ut pal (Himalayan poppy)	
ba le ka (birthwort)	
tig ta (chiretta)	
brag zhun (mineral pitch)	
ru rta (costus)	Reduce fever while also supporting the digestive system
ba sha ka (Malabar nut tree)	
gser gyi me tog (bolenggua)	

Treats inflammation and enlargement of the liver caused by dark phlegm.

tig ta 8

Chiretta 8

tig ta (chiretta)	Treat bile-related fever
gser gyi me tog (bolenggua)	
bong nga dkar po (white aconite)	
ru rta (costus)	Supports the digestive system

par pa ta (fumitory)	
hong len (picrorhiza grass)	Treat fever
rtsa mkhris (rabbit milkweed)	
skyer pa'i bar shun (barberry root middle bark)	

Treats fever with inflammation and bile disorders.

tig ta 25

Chiretta 25

rgya tig (Indian chiretta)	Three Bitters; lower bile, blood, liver, and gallbladder fever
bal tig (Nepalese chiretta)	
bod tig (Tibetan chiretta)	
gser gyi me tog (bolenggua)	Treat bile
dug mo nyung (kurchi)	
rgun 'brum (raisin)	
kyi lce (broad-leaf gentian)	
bong nga dkar po (white aconite)	
dzA ti (nutmeg)	Protect the seven bodily constituents and rejuvenate
a ru ra (chebulic myrobalan)	
ru rta (costus)	
cu gang (bamboo pith)	Treat fever
brag zhun (mineral pitch)	
ba sha ka (Malabar nut tree)	
se 'bru (pomegranate)	Pomegranate Combination; protects the stomach from the damaging effects of cold herbs
gur gum (safflower)	
sug smel (green cardamom)	
pi pi ling (long pepper)	
dom mkhris (bear bile)	Helps heal tissue injured by heat

li shi (clove)	Supports the digestive system and prevents increase of the wind humor
seng ldeng (catechu tree)	Treats fever
thang phrom (nightshade)	Treats infection
a krong (sandwort)	Treats lung fever
rgya skyegs (shellac)	Remove heat from the kidneys
shug pa tsher can (juniper)	

Treats bile disorders; this is a very general formula.

tsan dan 18

Sandalwood 18

tsan dan dkar po (white sandalwood)	Two Sandalwoods treat fever
tsan dan dmar po (red sandalwood)	
gi waM (elephant or ox gallstone)	Treats fever
cu gang (bamboo pith)	Six Excellent Drugs; balance the three humors and benefit the six internal organs
dzA ti (nutmeg)	
li shi (clove)	
ka ko la (black cardamom)	
gur gum (safflower)	
sug smel (green cardamom)	
a ru ra (chebulic myrobalan)	Treat fever
sum cu tig (Lhasa saxifrage)	
ru rta (costus)	
pri yang ku (nodding dragonhead)	

hong len (picrorhiza grass)	
re skon (Nepalese fumewort)	
ba sha ka (Malabar nut tree)	Cool the blood
'bri mog (groomwell)	
btsod (Indian madder)	

- Harmonizes the wind humor at its various natural locations.
- Treats inflammation of the liver, gallbladder, stomach, and intestines.
- Relieves diarrhea, intestinal spasms, and vomiting.
- Relieves pain in the ribs and upper back.
- Treats blockage of wind in the heart.
- Dissipates nodules caused by excessive strain (e.g. repetitive motion injury).
- Treats headache and blurred vision.
- This formula is given as a powder with a decoction of *brag zhun* (mineral pitch).

Formulas That Treat Blood and Lymph Disorders

spos dkar 10

Frankincense 10

spos dkar (frankincense)	Treats lymph (*chu ser*) disorders
a ru ra (chebulic myrobalan)	Three Fruits; treat fever
ba ru ra (beleric myrobalan)	
skyu ru ra (amla)	
thal ka rdo rje (foetid cassia)	Lymph Three (with frankincense above); treat lymph (*chu ser*) disorders
so ma rA dza (aibika)	
ru rta (costus)	Treats blood disorders
sle tres (moonseed)	Treats arthritis
ba sha ka (Malabar nut tree)	Treats blood disorders
brag zhun (mineral pitch)	Balances the three humors

- Treats blood and lymph (*chu ser*) disorders.
- Treats arthritis of the extremities.
- Treats skin eruptions.

klu bdud 18

Bellflower 18

klu bdud rdo rje (bonnet bellflower)	Treats lymph (*chu ser*) disorders
bong nga nag po (dark-blue aconite)	Alleviates pain
thal ka rdo rje (foetid cassia)	Treats lymph (*chu ser*) disorders
stong ri zil pa (fumewort)	Reduce fever
brag zhun (mineral pitch)	
shu dag nag po (sweet flag)	
sle tres (moonseed)	

a ru ra (chebulic myrobalan)	Balance the humors and support the seven bodily constituents
dbang po lag pa (salep orchid)	
ba ru ra (beleric myrobalan)	
spos dkar (frankincense)	Treat lymph *(chu ser)* disorders
gla rtsi (musk)	
so ma rA dza (aibika)	
gu gul (myrrh)	
seng ldeng (catechu tree)	
ba sha ka (Malabar nut tree)	Cool the blood
skyu ru ra (amla)	
ru rta (costus)	

- Treats hot lymph *(chu ser)* disorders.
- Treats gout and arthritis.
- Treats sinusitis, abscesses, elephantiasis, itching, leprosy, and other skin disorders.
- Relieves inflammation and pain.

Formulas That Treat Phlegm Disorders and Impaired Digestion

gar nag 10

Black Camphor 10

se 'bru (pomegranate)	Pomegranate Combination; warms the stomach and improves digestion
shing tsha (cinnamon)	
sug smel (green cardamom)	
pi pi ling (long pepper)	
a ru ra (chebulic myrobalan)	Balances the humors
rgyam tshwa (rock salt)	Treats indigestion
gser gyi me tog (bolenggua)	Treat bile
dug mo nyung (kurchi)	
dom mkhris (bear bile)	Helps protect and heal the intestines
gar nag (calcined wild-boar stool)	Supports the digestive system while balancing the warming effects of the other herbs in the formula

- Treats cold-bile disorders.
- Improves digestion.
- Treats hepatitis.

cong zhi 6

Calcite 6

se 'bru (pomegranate)	Treat phlegm and increase digestive heat
cong zhi (calcite)	
sug smel (green cardamom)	
pi pi ling (long pepper)	
ru rta (costus)	

| *gur gum* (safflower) | Directs the formula to the liver and thus treats acid reflux |

- Treats phlegm-related heartburn.
- Relieves acid reflux.

se 'bru nyi ma'i dkyil 'khor

Sun Mandala with Pomegranate

se 'bru (pomegranate)	
shing tsha (cinnamon)	Pomegranate Combination; warms the stomach and improves digestion
pi pi ling (long pepper)	
sug smel (green cardamom)	
gur gum (safflower)	
lcam pa (mallow)	Alleviates urinary blockage
lca ba (angelica)	
ra mnye (Solomon's seal)	Five Roots; increase digestion, physical vigor, and kidney heat
gze ma (puncture vine)	
ba spru (Himalayan mirabilis)	
nye shing (asparagus)	
sbrang rtsi (honey)	Treats phlegm

- Treats impaired digestion.
- Dissolves tumors.
- Treats early-stage edema (skya bab).

dwa lis 16

Rhododendron 16

se 'bru (pomegranate)	Pomegranate Sanctuary; helps the assimilation of nutrients by increasing the digestive heat
shing tsha (cinnamon)	
pi pi ling (long pepper)	
sug smel (green cardamom)	
gur gum (safflower)	
ru rta (costus)	Relieve miscellaneous wind disorders
li shi (clove)	
a ga ru (eaglewood)	
dzA ti (nutmeg)	
snying zho sha (lapsi tree)	
rgun 'brum (raisin)	Help the lungs eliminate lymph (*chu ser*) and edema
cu gang (bamboo pith)	
shing mngar (licorice)	
li ga dur (cranesbill)	
dwa lis (rhododendron)	
sdig srin (crab)	

- Treats impaired digestion and abdominal spasms.
- Benefits conditions where both heat and cold are present in the body and fighting.
- Relieves stiffness of the shoulders and upper back.
- Treats dizziness and vertigo caused by phlegm and wind.
- Treats cough and loss of voice.
- Relieves anemia (*skya rbab*).
- Treats swelling of the entire body.

Remark

Another formula by the same name but for different indications contains the following ingredients: *dwa lis* (rhododendron), *se 'bru* (pomegranate), *pi pi ling* (long pepper), *li shi* (clove), *snying zho sha* (lapsi tree), *shing mngar* (licorice), *cu gang* (bamboo pith), *ru rta* (costus), *rgun 'brum* (raisin), *a ga ru* (eaglewood), *sug smel* (green cardamom), *gur gum* (safflower), *dzA ti* (nutmeg), *shing tsha* (cinnamon), *li ga dur* (cranesbill), and *sdig srin* (crab).

se 'bru 5

Pomegranate 5

se 'bru (pomegranate)	Pomegranate Four; increase digestive heat
shing tsha (cinnamon)	
sug smel (green cardamom)	
sga skya (galangal)	
pi pi ling (long pepper)	Warms the spleen

Increases stomach heat, warms the extremities, and relieves lumbar pain.

Formulas That Treat Dark-phlegm Disorders

grub thob ril dkar

Thangtong Gyalpo's White Pill

It is said that this formula was revealed to Thangtong Gyalpo (*thang stong rgyal po*, 14th–15th centuries CE) by *dakinis*[21] while he was meditating (Tsewang Tsarong 1986).

a ru ra (chebulic myrobalan)	Balances the humors
hong len (picrorhiza grass)	Treats bile and blood
cong zhi (calcite)	Treats phlegm
re skon (Nepalese fumewort)	Treats fever in the channels
kham bu (apricot kernel)	Dries lymph *(chu ser)*
brag zhun (mineral pitch)	Balances the humors and rejuvenates

- Is beneficial for all minor disorders, internal and external, including those caused by spirits.
- Treats phlegm and blood disorders.

cong zhi 21

Calcite 21

cong zhi (calcite)	
ba sha ka (Malabar nut tree)	
se 'bru (pomegranate)	
sug smel (green cardamom)	
dug mo nyung (kurchi)	Treat dark phlegm
pri yang ku (nodding dragonhead)	
ru rta (costus)	
a ru ra (chebulic myrobalan)	

[21.] See the chapter on epidemic fever.

na le sham (black pepper)	Treat phlegm and fever and support the digestive system
gser gyi me tog (bolenggua)	
bong nga dkar po (white aconite)	Treat bile- and blood-related fever and dark phlegm
ma nu pa tra (elecampane)	
ut pal (Himalayan poppy)	
tig ta (chiretta)	
tsan dan dmar po (red sandalwood)	
bse yab (Chinese quince)	
brag zhun (mineral pitch)	
skyu ru ra (amla)	
gi waM (elephant or ox gallstone)	Treats fever and poisoning
star bu (sea buckthorn)	Treat dark phlegm
'u su (coriander)	

Treats dark phlegm accompanied by sour and watery vomitus, stomach pain, and dry feces.

thang chen 25

Great Decoction 25

kha che gur gum (saffron)	Treats fever in the channels
a ru ra (chebulic myrobalan)	Three Fruits; gather and treat fever, rejuvenate, balance the humors
ba ru ra (beleric myrobalan)	
skyu ru ra (amla)	
ma nu pa tra (elecampane)	Treat phlegm and fever
pu Shkara mU la (Himalayan elecampane)	
tig ta (chiretta)	Treat blood and bile
hong len (picrorhiza grass)	

kyi lce (broad-leaf gentian)	Treat bile and fever
bong nga dkar po (white aconite)	
'u su (coriander)	
par pa ta (fumitory)	
a byag gzer 'joms (Tartar chrysanthemum)	
dbyi mong (clematis)	Treat fever and bile and support the digestive system
gser gyi me tog (bolenggua)	
ldum bu re ral (fern)	
phag khrag (pig's blood)	Detoxify and prevent wind and dark phlegm
gang gA chung (Gentiana urnula)	
ut pal (Himalayan poppy)	
ba sha ka (Malabar nut tree)	
pri yang ku (nodding dragonhead)	
brag zhun (mineral pitch)	
se 'bru (pomegranate)	Support the digestive system and prevent wind, phlegm, and dark phlegm
sug smel (green cardamom)	
bse yab (Chinese quince)	

- Gathers scattered fever, especially chronic fever or fever associated with dark phlegm or compounded poisons.
- Treats bile and phlegm disorders without increasing wind.
- Balances heat and cold in the body.
- Increases the appetite.

bde byed snyoms ldan

Balancing Comforter

cong zhi (calcite)	Treat phlegm
se 'bru (pomegranate)	
cu gang (bamboo pith)	Six Excellent Drugs; balance the three humors and benefit the six internal organs
gur gum (safflower)	
li shi (clove)	
dzA ti (nutmeg)	
sug smel (green cardamom)	
ka ko la (black cardamom)	
a ru ra (chebulic myrobalan)	Balance the three humors and support the digestive system
shing tsha (cinnamon)	
dwa lis (rhododendron)	

Treats phlegm disorders combined with either wind or bile, especially if the digestive power of the spleen is weakened, if there is a lymph *(chu ser)* disorder, or if there is a skin disorder.

bde myug

Seed of Comfort

cu gang (bamboo pith)	Treat dark phlegm
skyu ru ra (amla)	
brag zhun (mineral pitch)	
rgyam tshwa (rock salt)	
gur gum (safflower)	Regulate the menses and benefit the liver
sbrul gyi sha (processed snake meat)	

sug smel (green cardamom)	Balance the humors and support the seven bodily constituents
a ru ra (chebulic myrobalan)	
ru rta (costus)	
pi pi ling (long pepper)	
'u su (coriander)	
se 'bru (pomegranate)	
ba sha ka (Malabar nut tree)	Treat dark phlegm and poisoning
star bu (sea buckthorn)	
pu Shkara mU la (Himalayan elecampane)	
ut pal (Himalayan poppy)	
lcags (iron)	

Treats dark phlegm accompanied by pain, vomiting, or sour watery fluid; or by blood, indigestion, dysmenorrhea, or irregular menses.

man ngag bsil sbyor

Cooling Preparation from the Secret Oral Tradition

tsan dan dkar po (white sandalwood)	Three Precious Woods; treat fever and wind Two Sandalwoods
tsan dan dmar po (red sandalwood)	
a ga ru (eaglewood)	
gi waM (elephant or ox gallstone)	Treat fever and benefit the liver and spleen
ut pal (Himalayan poppy)	
gser gyi me tog (bolenggua)	
a ru ra (chebulic myrobalan)	
sug smel (green cardamom)	Six Excellent Drugs; balance the three humors and benefit the six internal organs
ka ko la (black cardamom)	
li shi (clove)	
gur gum (safflower)	
dzA ti (nutmeg)	
cu gang (bamboo pith)	

bong nga dkar po (white aconite)	Treat bile
gla rtsi (musk)	
dug mo nyung (kurchi)	
pi pi ling (long pepper)	Treat dark phlegm
ru rta (costus)	
tig ta (chiretta)	
pri yang ku (nodding dragonhead)	
ba sha ka (Malabar nut tree)	
se 'bru (pomegranate)	Treat phlegm
skyu ru ra (amla)	
cong zhi (calcite)	

- Treats dark phlegm.
- Treats poisoning.
- Treats blood disorders.
- Treats fever associated with phlegm.
- Benefits the spleen and the liver.

g.yu dril 13

Turquoise Concentrate 13

ru rta (costus)	Balance the humors and treat dark phlegm
skyu ru ra (amla)	
se 'bru (pomegranate)	
ba sha ka (Malabar nut tree)	
sug smel (green cardamom)	Support the digestive system
pi pi ling (long pepper)	
pri yang ku (nodding dragonhead)	Treat dark phlegm
'u su (coriander)	
ut pal (Himalayan poppy)	Treats fever
re skon (Nepalese fumewort)	Treats fever and dark phlegm

bca 'sga (fresh ginger)	Support the digestive heat
go thal (calcined caraway)	
byi tang ga (false black pepper)	

- Treats dark phlegm, especially when both heat and cold are present and fighting each other.
- Treats colic and impaired indigestion and expels worms.
- Helps certain gynecological disorders.

ru rta 6

Costus 6

ru rta (costus)	Treat dark phlegm
skyu ru ra (amla)	
se 'bru (pomegranate)	
ba sha ka (Malabar nut tree)	
sug smel (green cardamom)	Support the digestive system
pi pi ling (long pepper)	

- Treats dark phlegm.
- Alleviates various digestive problems such as colic, eructation, gastritis, nausea, vomiting, and flatulence.

Formulas That Treat Contagious Disorders, Fever, and Inflammation

khyung 5

Garuda 5

This formula's origin is attributed to the following legend: There was once a kingdom in eastern India whose inhabitants were bothered by lymph *(chu ser)* disorders and diseases caused by *klu* (subterranean or aquatic elemental spirits) and by microorganisms; it was possibly leprosy. Not knowing where to turn, the king and his subjects took refuge in the Three Jewels (Buddha, dharma, and sangha). As a result of this observance, Garuda (a mythical bird) manifested to help the kingdom and cleared away the obstacles faced by the people. When he was about to die, Garuda offered his body as medicine so that the people could continue to enjoy his blessings in the form of pills to be taken internally or worn as amulets. Garuda further promised that when the materials of his body were exhausted, his blessings would continue in the form of drugs. Thus it is said that *a ru ra* (chebulic myrobalan) symbolizes Garuda's flesh, *ru rta* (costus) symbolizes Garuda's bones, *shu dag nag po* (sweet flag) symbolizes Garuda's muscles, *gla rtsi* (musk) symbolizes Garuda's blood, and *bong nga nag po* (dark-blue aconite) symbolizes Garuda's heart.

a ru ra (chebulic myrobalan)	Treats all ailments and balances the humors
ru rta (costus)	Treats wind and bile and benefits the stomach
shu dag nag po (sweet flag)	Treats wind and contagious fever and supports the digestive system
gla rtsi (musk)	Treats infectious disorders
bong nga nag po (dark-blue aconite)	Alleviates pain and inflammation

- Treats leprosy and lymph *(chu ser)* disorders.
- Treats inflammation of the head, ears, nose, and gums.
- Treats tonsillitis.
- Alleviates severe stomach pain and pain caused by intestinal parasites.
- Relieves itching and skin eruptions.

'khrug glo kun sel

Remover of All Lung Imbalances

spang rtsi do bo (Pterocephalus hookeri)	Treat lung fever
ba le ka (birthwort)	
a ru ra (chebulic myrobalan)	Three Fruits; treat fever
ba ru ra (beleric myrobalan)	
skyu ru ra (amla)	
ma nu pa tra (elecampane)	Treat infectious fever
ru rta (costus)	
cu gang (bamboo pith)	Treat lung fever
sro lo dkar po (Pegaeophyton scapiflorum)	
li ga dur (cranesbill)	
rgya skyegs (shellac)	Three Reds; treat fever in the blood and in the lungs
btsod (Indian madder)	
'bri mog (groomwell)	

- Treats spread fever.
- Treats blood disorders associated with wind.
- Treats chronic productive cough.
- Treats influenza that affects the lungs.

ga bur 25

Camphor 25

This formula is the basis for the modern variant commercialized as Padma 28 or Padma Basic.

ga bur (camphor)	Removes deep-rooted fever.
cu gang (bamboo pith)	Six Excellent Drugs; balance the three humors and benefit the six internal organs
kha che gur gum (saffron)	
li shi (clove)	
dzA ti (nutmeg)	
sug smel (green cardamom)	
ka ko la (black cardamom)	
a ga ru (eaglewood)	Three Precious Woods; treat fever and wind
tsan dan dkar po (white sandalwood)	
tsan dan dmar po (red sandalwood)	
ut pal (Himalayan poppy)	Treat fever
pad ma ge sar (silk cotton tree)	
nA ga ge sar (silk cotton tree)	
ru rta (costus)	Treat fever and support the digestive system
zi ra dkar po (cumin)	
ba le ka (birthwort)	
shing tsha (cinnamon)	
chu srin sder mo (spike moss)	
pu shel rtse (noble dendrobium)	
spang spos (muskroot)	
rdo dreg (salted shield)	Benefit the lungs
'bu su hang (alfalfa)	

a ru ra (chebulic myrobalan)	Three Fruits; treat fever, rejuvenate, balance the three humors
ba ru ra (beleric myrobalan)	
skyu ru ra (amla)	

- Treats all types of fever, especially chronic fever.
- Treats arthritis.
- Treats *me dbal* ("fire blotch"), an inflammatory skin disorder.

gur gum 13

Safflower 13

gur gum (safflower)	Treat fever in the channels
li shi (clove)	
gi waM (elephant or ox gallstone)	Treat fever, wind, and blood; cool the liver
bse ru'i rwa (rhinoceros horn)	
mtshal (cinnabar)	
tsan dan dkar po (white sandalwood)	
gla rtsi (musk)	
'jam 'bras (fever nut)	Warms the kidneys
bong nga dkar po (white aconite)	Treats fever
ru rta (costus)	Supports the digestive system
a ru ra (chebulic myrobalan)	Three Fruits; treat fever and rejuvenate
ba ru ra (beleric myrobalan)	
skyu ru ra (amla)	

- Benefits the liver.
- Heals trauma of the kidneys.
- Helps difficult urination.
- Treats sinusitis.

cu gang 25

Bamboo Pith 25

cu gang (bamboo pith)	Six Excellent Drugs; balance the three humors and benefit the six internal organs
dzA ti (nutmeg)	
li shi (clove)	
gur gum (safflower)	
sug smel (green cardamom)	
ka ko la (black cardamom)	
gi waM (elephant or ox gallstone)	Treats inflammation
shing mngar (licorice)	Benefit the lungs
rgun 'brum (raisin)	
sro lo dmar po (rhodiola)	
mkhan pa a krong (Ajania sp.)	Treat lung fever and remove pus and phlegm
star bu (sea buckthorn)	
ru rta (costus)	
li ga dur (cranesbill)	
ba le ka (birthwort)	
hong len (picrorhiza grass)	Treats inflammation
tsan dan dkar po (white sandalwood)	Two Sandalwoods; treat fever
tsan dan dmar po (red sandalwood)	
a ru ra (chebulic myrobalan)	Three Fruits; treat fever and rejuvenate
ba ru ra (beleric myrobalan)	
skyu ru ra (amla)	
pa yag rtsa ba (Tibetan lancea)	Remove mucus and pus from the lungs and treat lung fever
a krong (sandwort)	
tshar bong rtsa ba (artemisia root)	
zi ra dkar po (cumin)	Supports the digestive system

Treats acute or chronic lung fever accompanied by chest pain, bloody sputum, cough, inflammation, dyspnea, cold sweating, weight loss, and fatigue.

star bu 5

Sea Buckthorn 5

star bu (sea buckthorn)	Removes phlegm from the lungs
shing mngar (licorice)	Opens the channels and cools the lungs
rgun 'brum (raisin)	Purges fever from the lungs
skyu ru ra (amla)	Treats blood, bile, and phlegm
ru rta (costus)	Cools the blood and bile and supports the digestive system

- Treats chronic inflammation of the lungs.
- Treats hidden and void fevers.
- Expels pus and blood from the lungs and alleviates cough.

nor bu bdun thang

Decoction of Seven Precious Ingredients

ma nu pa tra (elecampane)	Elecampane Four; treat recently acquired fever
kaNDa ka ri (two-flowered raspberry)	
sle tres (moonseed)	
sga skya (galangal)	
a ru ra (chebulic myrobalan)	Three Fruits; ripen and treat fever and protect the bodily constituents
ba ru ra (beleric myrobalan)	
skyu ru ra (amla)	

- Treats fever associated with wind that threatens the seven bodily constituents.
- Treats and prevents the common cold.
- Ripens fever.
- Prevents minor fevers from spreading.

spang rgyan 15

Gentian 15

spang rgyan (small-leaf gentian)	Treat fever of the heart and lungs
a ga ru (eaglewood)	
snying zho sha (lapsi tree)	
tsan dan dkar po (white sandalwood)	
dzA ti (nutmeg)	
cu gang (bamboo pith)	
sro lo dkar po (Pegaeophyton scapiflorum)	
gur gum (safflower)	Benefits the eyes by directing the action of the formula to the liver
a ru ra (chebulic myrobalan)	Three Fruits; treat fever and rejuvenate
ba ru ra (beleric myrobalan)	
skyu ru ra (amla)	
sle tres (moonseed)	Treat fever, wind, and blood
ba sha ka (Malabar nut tree)	
li shi (clove)	
ru rta (costus)	
shing mngar (licorice)	Benefits the lungs

- Treats inflammations of the lungs and alleviates asthma, sputum, cough, shortness of breath, hoarseness, and blood in the sputum.
- Benefits the eyes.

spang rtsi 12

Pterocephalus 12

spang rtsi do bo (Pterocephalus hookeri)	Treats infectious fever
bong nga dkar po (white aconite)	Treats bile fever
stag sha (locoweed)	Treat epidemic fever
par pa ta (fumitory)	

bong nga nag po (dark-blue aconite)	Relieves pain
cu gang (bamboo pith)	Treat fever
gur gum (safflower)	
gi waM (elephant or ox gallstone)	
tsan dan dkar po (white sandalwood)	
brag zhun (mineral pitch)	
gla rtsi (musk)	
gu gul (myrrh)	

Treats fever associated with inflammation and severe infections.

phan pa kun ldan

All–Beneficial

thang phrom (nightshade)	Treat infectious fever and inflammation, dispel toxins, and alleviate pain
gu gul (myrrh)	
'dzin pa (blue aconite)	
a ru ra (chebulic myrobalan)	
yung ba (turmeric)	
stag sha (locoweed)	
shu dag nag po (sweet flag)	
rgya tshwa (ammonium chloride)	
ma ru rtse (flame of the forest)	Treat phlegm
byi tang ga (false pepper)	
bong nga nag po (dark-blue aconite)	Alleviates pain

- Treats inflammation, muscle pain, and contagious disorders.
- Treats sinusitis.
- Treats swelling of the tongue, gums, and palate.
- Brings pus to the surface to facilitate the healing of sores.

gtso bo 8

Principal 8

gi waM (elephant or ox gallstone)	Treat fever
tsan dan dkar po (white sandalwood)	
cu gang (bamboo pith)	
gur gum (safflower)	
tig ta (chiretta)	Treat blood and bile
ba sha ka (Malabar nut tree)	
hong len (picrorhiza grass)	
bong nga dkar po (white aconite)	Treats bile fever

Treats chronic spread fever with symptoms such as thirst, a bitter taste in the mouth, cough, and pain in the vertebrae.

gtso bo 25

Principal 25

gi waM (elephant or ox gallstone)	Principal Eight
tsan dan dkar po (white sandalwood)	
cu gang (bamboo pith)	
gur gum (safflower)	
tig ta (chiretta)	
ba sha ka (Malabar nut tree)	
hong len (picrorhiza grass)	
bong nga dkar po (white aconite)	
a 'bras (mango)	Three Seeds; warm the kidneys
sra 'bras (Java plum)	
'jam 'bras (fever nut)	

ma nu pa tra (elecampane)	Elecampane Four; treat recently acquired fever
sle tres (moonseed)	
kaNDa ka ri (two-flowered raspberry)	
sga skya (galangal)	
star bu (sea buckthorn)	Treat lung fever
rgun 'brum (raisin)	
li ga dur (cranesbill)	
shing mngar (licorice)	
spang rgyan (small-leaf gentian)	
pa yag rtsa ba (Tibetan lancea)	
a krong (sandwort)	
wa yi glo ba (lung of fox or other large animal)	
zi ra dkar po (cumin)	Support the digestive system
bong nga nag po (dark-blue aconite)	

- Treats major and minor inflammatory fever conditions, especially those that affect the lungs and the bones.
- Relieves cough, panting, shortness of breath, fainting, nausea, and insomnia.

li shi 6

Clove 6

li shi mtshon 'khor (star anise)	Treat fever of the throat and lungs
cu gang (bamboo pith)	
shing mngar (licorice)	
spang rgyan (small-leaf gentian)	
ru rta (costus)	Supports the digestive system and treats disturbed fever
a ru ra (chebulic myrobalan)	Balances the humors, treats infections, and detoxifies

- Treats fever, especially toxic fever.
- Relieves inflammation of the lungs, throat, and neck.
- Relieves cough and hoarseness.

Formulas That Treat Disorders of the Internal Organs

rgun 'brum 7

Raisin 7

rgun 'brum (raisin)	Benefit the lungs
cu gang (bamboo pith)	
gur gum (safflower)	
shing mngar (licorice)	
gla sgang (bistort)	
shing tsha (cinnamon)	Support the digestive system
se 'bru (pomegranate)	

Benefits the lungs and alleviates cough and dyspnea.

rgwa lo ba'i sman mar

Galoba's Medicinal Butter

'bri mog (groomwell)	Treats lung fever
cong zhi (calcite)	Rejuvenates the lungs
ba sha ka (Malabar nut tree)	Cools the blood
shing mngar (licorice)	Benefits the lungs
ru rta (costus)	Treats fever and supports the digestive system

Treats phlegm and blood that affect the lungs.

bse ru 25

Rhinoceros 25

bse ru'i rwa (rhinoceros horn)	Treat lung disorders and remove pus, blood and edema
sha ru (deer horn)	
dzA ti (nutmeg)	Six Excellent Drugs, balance the three humors and benefit the six internal organs
li shi (clove)	
sug smel (green cardamom)	
cu gang (bamboo pith)	
ka ko la (black cardamom)	
gur gum (safflower)	
ru rta (costus)	Treats the blood
tsan dan dkar po (white sandalwood)	Two Sandalwoods, treat fever
tsan dan dmar po (red sandalwood)	
nA ga ge sar (silk cotton tree)	Remove heat from the lungs
pad ma ge sar (silk cotton tree)	
rgya ru (serow horn)	Helps blood circulation and detoxifies
thal ka rdo rje (foetid cassia)	Direct the formula to the lymph (*chu ser*)
so ma rA dza (aibika)	
go snyod (caraway)	Supports the digestive heat
ut pal (Himalayan poppy)	Treat fever and cool the blood
ba sha ka (Malabar nut tree)	
gi waM (elephant or ox gallstone)	
li ga dur (cranesbill)	
a ru ra (chebulic myrobalan)	
skyu ru ra (amla)	
star bu (sea buckthorn)	Benefit the lungs and cool fever
'bri mog (groomwell)	

Treats lung disorders in general and especially those with pus, blood, or lymph (*chu ser*).

a ru 7

Chebulic Myrobalan 7

a ru ra (chebulic myrobalan)	Harmonize the spleen
nA ga ge sar (silk cotton tree)	
li shi (clove)	
pi pi ling (long pepper)	
gser gyi me tog (bolenggua)	Reduce fever from the spleen and stomach
ka ko la (black cardamom)	
spang spos (muskroot)	

Treats injury or disturbance to the spleen resulting in fever, pain, and enlargement of the spleen.

Formulas That Expel Microbes and Parasites

'chi med srin sel

Unfailing Remover of Microorganisms

bong nga dkar po (white aconite)	Treats epidemic fever
a ru ra (chebulic myrobalan)	Treats infections
ru rta (costus)	Treats disturbed fever
shu dag nag po (sweet flag)	Treats contagious fever and supports the digestive system
gla rtsi (musk)	Treats infection and poisoning
byi tang ga (false black pepper)	Supports the digestive system and expels parasites

- Removes worms and parasites that cause either hot or cold conditions.
- Alleviates sudden pain caused by infectious diseases.

byi tang 7

False Black Pepper 7

byi tang ga (false black pepper)	Expel parasites
sgog skya (garlic)	
ma ru rtse (flame of the forest)	
so ma rA dza (aibika)	Relieves itching caused by lymph (*chu ser*)
gres ma (iris)	Expel parasites
phur thal (calcined *Artemisia sp.*)	
gla rtsi (musk)	

- Expels intestinal worms.
- Relieves anal itching.

Formulas That Treat Musculoskeletal and Paralytic Disorders

gur khyung phyag rdor can

Vajrapani–like Preparation

gur gum (safflower)	Safflower 13
li shi (clove)	
gi waM (elephant or ox gallstone)	
bse ru'i rwa (rhinoceros horn)	
mtshal (cinnabar)	
tsan dan dmar po (red sandalwood)	
gla rtsi (musk)	
'jam 'bras (fever nut)	
bong nga dkar po (white aconite)	
ru rta (costus)	
a ru ra (chebulic myrobalan)	
ba ru ra (beleric myrobalan)	
skyu ru ra (amla)	
lug mur (Phlomis younghusbandii)	Treat infectious fever
stag sha (locoweed)	
spos dkar (frankincense)	Lymph Three; treat lymph *(chu ser)* disorders
thal ka rdo rje (foetid cassia)	
so ma rA dza (aibika)	
seng ldeng (catechu tree)	Treats blood and lymph *(chu ser)*

bong nga nag po (dark-blue aconite)	Relieve joint pain
gu gul (myrrh)	
shu dag nag po (sweet flag)	Treats wind and balances the bodily constituents

- Treats infections, including nephritis and rhinitis.
- Treats arthritis.
- Treats paralysis due to stroke.
- Treats leprosy.

dwa lis 18

Rhododendron 18

dwa lis (rhododendron)	Empirical hypotensive, bradycardic, and analgesic
kyi lce (broad-leaf gentian)	
shing mngar (licorice)	Treats channel disorders
dzA ti (nutmeg)	
li shi (clove)	
cu gang (bamboo pith)	Six Excellent Drugs; balance the three humors and benefit the six internal organs
gur gum (safflower)	
sug smel (green cardamom)	
ka ko la (black cardamom)	
tsan dan dkar po (white sandalwood)	
tsan dan dmar po (red sandalwood)	Three Precious Woods; treat fever and wind
a ga ru (eaglewood)	
a ru ra (chebulic myrobalan)	
ba ru ra (beleric myrobalan)	Three Fruits; balance the three humors
skyu ru ra (amla)	

rgya skyegs (shellac)	Three Reds; treat fever in the blood and in the lungs and remove heat from the kidneys
btsod (Indian madder)	
zhu mkhan (sapphireberry)	

Treats paralysis, Parkinsonism, and other nervous disorders.

Remark

Another formula by the same name but for different indications contains the following ingredients: *dwa lis* (rhododendron), *ka ko la* (black cardamom), *a ru ra* (chebulic myrobalan), *tsan dan dkar po* (white sandalwood), *ba ru ra* (beleric myrobalan), *tsan dan dmar po* (red sandalwood), *skyu ru ra* (amla), *zhu mkhan* (sapphireberry), *cu gang* (bamboo pith), *btsod* (Indian madder), *gur gum* (safflower), *mtshal* (cinnabar), *dzA ti* (nutmeg), *kyi lce* (broad-leaf gentian), *li shi* (clove), *shing tsha* (cinnamon), *sug smel* (green cardamom), and *a ga ru* (eaglewood).

sle tres lnga thang

Moonseed 5 Decoction

sle tres (moonseed)	Treats arthritis
a ru ra (chebulic myrobalan)	Three Fruits; treat fever
ba ru ra (beleric myrobalan)	
skyu ru ra (amla)	
tig ta (chiretta)	Cools the blood

- Treats blood and lymph *(chu ser)* disorders.
- Treats arthritis.

bsam 'phel nor bu

Wish-fulfilling Jewel

cu gang (bamboo pith)	Six Excellent Drugs; balance the three humors and benefit the six internal organs
gur gum (safflower)	
li shi (clove)	
dzA ti (nutmeg)	
sug smel (green cardamom)	
ka ko la (black cardamom)	
tsan dan dkar po (white sandalwood)	Three Precious Woods; treat fever and wind
tsan dan dmar po (red sandalwood)	
a ga ru (eaglewood)	
gla rtsi (musk)	Benefit the channels
gi waM (elephant or ox gallstone)	
mu tig (pearl)	Treat poisoning
bse ru'i rwa (rhinoceros horn)	
a ru ra (chebulic myrobalan)	Three Fruits; treat fever and rejuvenate
ba ru ra (beleric myrobalan)	
skyu ru ra (amla)	
zi ra dkar po (cumin)	Two Cumins; benefit the stomach
zi ra nag po (fennelflower)	
spos dkar (frankincense)	Lymph Three; treat lymph (*chu ser*) disorders
thal ka rdo rje (foetid cassia)	
so ma rA dza (aibika)	
pi pi ling (long pepper)	Support the spleen
sman sga (ginger)	
shing tsha (cinnamon)	
ma nu pa tra (elecampane)	Treat wind and blood
ru rta (costus)	

shing mngar (licorice)	
lcam pa (mallow)	Benefit the channels
'bri rta sa 'dzin (wild strawberry)	
sdig srin (crab)	

- Treats inflammation of the channels and blood vessels.
- Benefits the brain and the spinal cord.
- Treats lymph *(chu ser)* disorders and gout.
- Treats "bending" and "flaccid" disorders such as contraction or flaccidity of the limbs, mouth and eye deviation, malfunction of the senses, etc.
- Treats pain in the lumbar area, hips, and spine.

Formulas That Treat Genitourinary and Degenerative Disorders

go yu 28

Betel Nut 28

se 'bru (pomegranate)	Pomegranate Combination; warms the stomach
shing tsha (cinnamon)	
pi pi ling (long pepper)	
sug smel (green cardamom)	
dong gra (lesser galangal)	Warms the stomach
gser gyis bye ma (vermiculite)	Warm the kidneys
bre ga (pennycress)	
a 'bras (mango)	Three Seeds; warm the kidneys
sra 'bras (Java plum)	
'jam 'bras (fever nut)	
rgya skyegs (shellac)	Three Reds; remove heat from the kidneys
btsod (Indian madder)	
zhu mkhan (sapphireberry)	
gla rtsi (musk)	Remove heat from the kidneys
mkhal ma zho sha (sword bean)	
ut pal (Himalayan poppy)	
shug pa tsher can (juniper)	
a ru ra (chebulic myrobalan)	Cool fever
gser gyi me tog (bolenggua)	
ba sha ka (Malabar nut tree)	
gze ma (puncture vine)	Benefit the urinary system
sdig srin (crab)	
pri yang ku (nodding dragonhead)	
lcam pa (mallow)	

skyer pa'i bar shun (barberry root middle bark)	Detoxify
brag zhun (mineral pitch)	
yung ba (turmeric)	
go yu (betel nut)	Benefits the kidneys

- Treats pelvic disorders, including pain, swollen testicles, kidney disorders, leukorrhea, irregular menses, and spermatorrhea.
- Restores kidney heat and alleviates lower back pain.

rgya ru 14

Serow Horn 14

rgya ru (serow horn)	Improve the flow of blood
bse ru'i rwa (rhinoceros horn)	
sha ru (deer horn)	
gur gum (safflower)	Open the channels
mtshal dkar (alum or massicot)	
dom mkhris (bear bile)	
tsan dan dmar po (red sandalwood)	Treat blood, wind, and phlegm
dzA ti (nutmeg)	
sug smel (green cardamom)	
rgya skyegs (shellac)	Remove heat from the kidneys and cool the blood
btsod (Indian madder)	
shug pa tsher can (juniper)	
se 'bru (pomegranate)	Warm the kidneys; guide formula to the uterus
ba spru (Himalayan mirabilis)	

- Regulates the flow of blood.
- Regulates the menses.
- Relieves pain in the lumbar, hip, and lower abdominal regions.

bre ga 13

Pennycress 13

bre ga (pennycress)	Treats urinary disorders
sra 'bras (Java plum)	Three Seeds; warm the kidneys
a 'bras (mango)	
'jam 'bras (fever nut)	
rgya skyegs (shellac)	Three Reds; remove heat from the kidneys
btsod (Indian madder)	
zhu mkhan (sapphireberry)	
shug pa tsher can (juniper)	Benefits the urinary system
a ru ra (chebulic myrobalan)	Rejuvenates and promotes diuresis
sug smel (green cardamom)	Warm the kidneys
mkhal ma zho sha (sword bean)	
ba sha ka (Malabar nut tree)	Reduces heat caused by inflammation

- Treats urinary disorders, especially ureteritis and urethritis.
- Relieves pain in the lumbar and pelvic areas.
- Reduces swelling of the knees and testicles.

'b'a sam sman mar

'b'a sam **Medicinal Butter**

a ru ra (chebulic myrobalan)	Three Fruits; balance the three humors (same total weight as the second group of herbs)
ba ru ra (beleric myrobalan)	
skyu ru ra (amla)	
lca ba (angelica)	Five Roots; increase digestion, physical vigor, and kidney heat (same total weight as the first group of herbs)
nye shing (asparagus)	
ra mnye (Solomon's seal)	
gze ma (puncture vine)	
ba spru (Himalayan mirabilis)	

Make as medicinal butter with milk and honey. When treating a cold disorder, the amount of the Five Roots should be greater than that of the Three Fruits, and vice versa for a hot disorder. This preparation tonifies and rejuvenates.

sug smel 10

Cardamom 10

sug smel (green cardamom)	Warms the kidneys
sga skya (galangal)	Support the warming action of *sug smel* (green cardamom)
rgyam tshwa (rock salt)	
pi pi ling (long pepper)	
gla rtsi (musk)	Benefit the urinary system
sdig srin (crab)	
lcam pa (mallow)	
a 'bras (mango)	Three Seeds; warm the kidneys
sra 'bras (Java plum)	
'jam 'bras (fever nut)	

Treats kidney disorders, especially kidney stones, urinary tumors, and other urinary blockages.

se 'bru kun bde

Universally Comforting Pomegranate

se 'bru (pomegranate)	Pomegranate Combination; warms the stomach and improves digestion
shing tsha (cinnamon)	
sug smel (green cardamom)	
pi pi ling (long pepper)	
gur gum (safflower)	
'u su (coriander)	Promotes digestive heat

hong len (picrorhiza grass)	
ba sha ka (Malabar nut tree)	
brag zhun (mineral pitch)	Benefit the liver and the blood
skyu ru ra (amla)	
sum cu tig (Lhasa saxifrage)	
bre ga (pennycress)	
lcam pa (mallow)	
sdig srin (crab)	Benefit the urinary system
pri yang ku (nodding dragonhead)	
spang rtsi do bo (*Pterocephalus hookeri*)	Eases lung congestion

- Increases stomach and kidney heat and alleviates pain in the lumbar area.
- Resolves swelling and congestion and eases breathing.

a ru 10

Chebulic Myrobalan 10

a ru ra (chebulic myrobalan)	Rejuvenates
gur gum (safflower)	Improves the circulation
sug smel (green cardamom)	
brag zhun (mineral pitch)	
tig ta (chiretta)	Reduce fever from the kidneys
mkhal ma zho sha (sword bean)	
zhu mkhan (sapphireberry)	
btsod (Indian madder)	Three Reds; remove heat from the kidneys
rgya skyegs (shellac)	
shug pa tsher can (juniper)	Reduces fever from the kidneys

Treats inflammation of the kidneys that causes pain in the lower part of the body and dribbling urine.

Miscellaneous Formulas

zhi byed 6

Pacifying 6

a ru ra (chebulic myrobalan)	Balances the humors and acts as a purgative
lcum rtsa (rhubarb)	Purgative
sga skya (galangal)	Support the digestive system
bul tog (soda ash)	
ma nu pa tra (elecampane)	
cong zhi (calcite)	Prevents diarrhea

Normalizes the purgative wind: treats disorders such as indigestion, flatulence, colic, constipation, difficult childbirth, and retained placenta.

a wa 15

Sedge 15

cong zhi (calcite)	Rejuvenate
cu gang (bamboo pith)	
gur gum (safflower)	Benefits the liver
ru rta (costus)	Supports the digestive system
gu gul (myrrh)	Benefits the liver
a ru ra (chebulic myrobalan)	Three Fruits; balance the three humors
ba ru ra (beleric myrobalan)	
skyu ru ra (amla)	
shing mngar (licorice)	Benefits the channels

sbrul mig (snake eyes)	
zi ra nag po (fennelflower)	
ut pal (Himalayan poppy)	Benefit the eyes
brag zhun (mineral pitch)	
lcags (iron)	
mdung rtsi (goethite)	

Benefits the eyes.

BLOODLETTING

Bloodletting is a strong heat-clearing modality of Tibetan medicine. It is typically used as a last-resort measure when other modalities have not been sufficient. This chapter is adapted from Chapter 20 of the Oral Instruction Tantra.

Benefits of Bloodletting

Bloodletting, when applied correctly, offers the following benefits:

- It alleviates disorders of the blood vessels and channels.
- It removes impure blood.
- It reduces swelling and pain.
- It removes sepsis at the root, for example in large pustules.
- It helps scars recover the complexion of normal skin.
- It helps reduce weight.

Bloodletting takes the real ailment and removes it through the blood. It is the most effective of the external therapies.

Indications and Contraindications

Suitable Ailments

Conditions amenable to bloodletting are disturbed fever, spread fever, epidemic fever, wound inflammation, gout, fiery *(me dbal)* skin disorders, burns, lymph *(chu ser)* disorders, leprosy, blood disorders, and bile disorders.

Contraindications

Even if one of the conditions above is present, there are strong contraindications to bloodletting therapy. These include elemental disturbance, emaciation, depletion of the seven bodily constituents, pregnancy, recent delivery, edema, consumptive disorders, lack of bodily heat, hemophilia, unripe epidemic fever, void fever, poisoning, inflammatory fever, and fever accompanied by weakness of the seven bodily constituents. In summary, bloodletting is contraindicated in phlegm and wind disorders. But if the patient's condition involves wind or phlegm in combination with bile, it may still be appropriate to perform bloodletting.

Bloodletting should not be performed on any of the patient's vulnerable points (one of the 45 points of the flesh, 8 points of the fat, 32 points of the bones, etc. as described in Chapter 4 of the Explanatory or Second Tantra), on the full moon, or on the new moon.

Bloodletting should not be performed on any of the *lha* points, i.e. points where the vital fluids are concentrated at a given day of the lunar cycle. It is customary to observe an extra day of safety margin; for example, no bloodletting should be performed on the new moon, full moon, or one day before or after either new or full moon. A lunar calendar should be consulted to ascertain the appropriateness of bloodletting specific points on a given day.

Indications

The diseases most suited to bloodletting are diseases of the blood above the diaphragm, continuous bleeding, fever when it is at its peak (fully developed fever), and disturbed fever.

Diseases fairly suited to bloodletting are:

- When there is shivering that stops after bloodletting has been done;
- When there is numbness or heaviness at the area considered for bloodletting;
- When the point to be bled bulges or is otherwise easy to find; and
- If the blood looks homogenous. If it does not look homogenous, it is best to treat the patient using herbs in order to separate the pure from the impure, using for example the Three Fruit decoction: *a ru ra* (chebulic myrobalan), *ba ru ra* (beleric myrobalan), and *skyu ru ra* (amla).

Blood and bile disorders when the impure blood has spread throughout the body are less suited for bloodletting, but may still be helped using appropriate clinical judgment.

The following cautions should be borne in mind:

- If the patient takes food that increases residual fever, the diet should be changed prior to performing bloodletting.
- If bloodletting is administered too early, this may stir up wind and cause fever to spread to the entire body.
- If bloodletting is administered too late, impure blood will disturb the channels and the impure blood will not be expelled. Instead, abscesses will form in the internal organs.

Technique

Instruments

The instruments used in bloodletting must be sharp and flexible. They must be made by a skilled blacksmith. (In practice, modern surgical implements such as lancets and scalpels certainly meet the criteria.) The doctor should carry this equipment wherever he or she goes.

Preparation

If there is hidden or unripe fever, it should be revealed or ripened. The ailment should be separated from the pure blood by giving the Three Fruit decoction. If the latter is not done, bloodletting will deplete the nutritive blood, wind will increase, and the fever will spread as a result.

At least half an hour before bloodletting, the patient should stay in the sun or near a source of heat. The environment should be calm, orderly, and free of disturbances so that treatment may proceed uninterrupted.

Palpation and Use of the Blade

If bloodletting is performed on an extremity, the limb should be tied proximally in order to reveal the vein. This technique is similar to modern phlebotomy and can be described in further detail in a clinical setting. The use of the blade is beyond the scope of this work.

Choice of Point

Chapter 20 of the Oral Instruction Tantra describes about 70 points suitable for bloodletting. The authors feel that precise description of the bloodletting points is best conveyed through oral instruction in the appropriate clinical setting.

Appearance of the Blood

When blood comes out, ideally its appearance should be consistent with the disease being treated. The blood should be fluid, thin, frothy, whitish, yellowish, or bluish and have some smell. This is a sign that the ailment will abate.

- If the blood is dark red and heterogeneous, herbal treatment is needed to separate the pure from the impure, as described above.
- If the blood looks very thin like pus, it is a sign of malnourishment. Rejuvenation therapy should be given before bloodletting can be done.

- If the blood is pale red, the treatment will not be beneficial unless a very small amount is drawn.
- Blood associated with bile disease appears yellowish and thin.
- Blood associated with phlegm disease appears smooth and pale red.
- Nutritive blood is the color of cinnabar (bright red) and should not be drawn.

Amount of Blood Drawn

If nutritive blood appears, this means that it is time to stop the bloodletting. But if the patient is very weak, the doctor should limit the amount of blood drawn (maybe a few ounces) without waiting for the appearance of nutritive blood.

- If there is strong pain in the internal organs, it may be desirable to draw even some of the nutritive blood.
- If there is nosebleed, this unchecked bleeding may be diverted by bleeding another appropriate location.
- If strong treatment is desired, it is best to draw less blood from several points. In all situations, the doctor should exercise sound clinical judgment.

Completion of Treatment

At the end of the treatment, the tie should be released and the area of the cut should be massaged gently. Afterward a cold stone should be applied followed by the appropriate bandage. The area of the cut should be kept protected.

Plum-Blossom Needle Treatment

The term "plum-blossom needle" is borrowed from traditional Chinese medicine. It describes a very light hammer whose head is mounted with needles. The hammer is tapped very gently on the patient's skin, just enough to make the skin bleed slightly. This technique is very effective in treating stiffness of the shoulder and is also employed to reduce toxic fever and chronic fever.

Complications

No Blood Coming Out

The blood may not come out for one of the following reasons:

- The patient's body is cold, possibly as a result of not staying warm prior to treatment.
- The instrument used for bleeding is blunt.

- The patient overate, thus blocking the channels and blood vessels.
- The patient is frightened.
- There are elemental disturbances.
- The treatment was disrupted.
- The cut is too small.
- The cut was not made correctly.
- The cut was made too early after tying the limb.
- The tie around the limb was released too soon.

No Diseased Blood Coming Out

If no diseased blood comes out, it is possible to try again at a nearby point, or to try again at the same point later during the day.

When the fever is almost gone, the blood vessels might be empty. This can make the drawing of impure blood more difficult. In that case, the following decoction may be given: *a ru ra* (chebulic myrobalan), *ba ru ra* (beleric myrobalan), *skyu ru ra* (amla), *ba le ka* (birthwort), *ut pal* (Himalayan poppy), *sle tres* (moonseed), *tig ta* (chiretta), *bong nga dkar po* (white aconite), *li ga dur* (cranesbill), and *ba sha ka* (Malabar nut tree).

Unchecked Bleeding

If bleeding does not stop, cold water should be sprinkled over the area. A cold water compress should be applied and tied into place. (Modern methods to stop bleeding require asepsis and the application of pressure.)

Swelling

The text describes several external treatments to reduce the swelling caused by bloodletting. This includes the powder of *rdo dreg* (salted shield), *spang spos* (musk-root), *gla sgang* (bistort), and *go snyod* (caraway) mixed with water into a poultice.

Fainting

Healing incense such as *spos dkar* (frankincense) should be burned near the patient together with *tsam pa* (roasted barley flour). The patient should then be given some animal blood to sip.

Increase of Wind

If wind increases as a result of bloodletting, this can normally be seen right away in signs such as yawning, stretching, etc. The patient should be given massage, *bu ram* (raw cane sugar) to suck on, wine made from *bu ram* (raw cane sugar), or noodle soup made with bones.

Iatrogenic Problems

Not Enough Blood Drawn

If an insufficient amount of blood is drawn, the disease will not be treated properly. This may cause tumors of the liver, dark phlegm, leprosy, cancer, skin blotches, accumulation of lymph *(chu ser)* in the chest and limbs, and pustules.

Too Much Blood Drawn

If too much blood is drawn, this will deplete the seven bodily constituents, increase the wind humor, and decrease the body heat and the digestive heat. This may lead to cold tumors, edema, or ascites.

Inappropriate Bloodletting

If bloodletting is applied to a condition that does not warrant it, e.g. a cold condition, the condition will be made worse.

Wrong Point or Technique

If the wrong point or the wrong technique is employed, there may be pain and local disturbance. A nerve may even be severed, with a resultant loss of sensation.

Moxibustion

The term moxibustion is derived from the Japanese name for mugwort, *mogusa* (艾), which is used in traditional Chinese, Japanese, and related healing systems. In these traditions, the heat of the burning herb is applied to acupuncture points or other specific locations of the body. The Tibetan practice refers to the application of strong heat, which is produced by burning a similar herb over specific points, sometimes to the point of leaving permanent scars. Historically, the practice of leaving scars after treatment has been found acceptable by its traditional client population. This chapter is adapted from Chapter 21 of the Oral Instruction Tantra.

Indications and Contraindications

Indications and Benefits

Moxibustion is beneficial for all phlegm, cold wind, channel, and lymph *(chu ser)* disorders. It is especially suited for impaired digestion *(ma zhu)*, decrease of the digestive fire, edema, ascites, tumors, cold-bile disorders, lymph *(chu ser)* disorders of the head or trunk, contagious diseases of the throat, void fever, all mental disorders, loss of consciousness, and all channel disorders.

Moxibustion offers the following benefits:

- It alleviates unbearable pain.
- It prevents the eruption of wind as a result of void fever or in the aftermath of any illness.
- It increases digestive fire and therefore helps digestion.
- It helps break tumors down.
- It helps heal chronic nonhealing sores.
- It stops the spread of malignant tumors.
- It reduces swelling caused by injury.
- It drains and dries lymph *(chu ser)* and prevents new lymph from forming.
- It protects the six hollow and five solid organs.
- It increases bodily heat and clears the mind.
- It prevents side effects from developing after other external therapies have been applied, especially bloodletting.
- It helps gather the disease, and thus can be used in hidden fever or unripe fever with the appropriate presentation.

Contraindications

- Moxibustion is contraindicated for all bile and blood disorders, but can be used for cold-bile disorders in some cases.
- Moxibustion should not be performed around the openings of the sense organs, i.e. eyes, ears, nose, or mouth.
- It should not be applied over the ovaries or testicles.
- One should not perform moxibustion over the vulnerable points of the body (one of the 45 points of the flesh, 8 points of the fat, 32 points of the bones, etc. as described in Chapter 4 of the Explanatory or Second Tantra), or over any other especially sensitive part.
- Moxibustion should not be performed on the 1st, 6th, 18th, 22nd, or 24th day of the lunar calendar or on the full moon.
- In autumn, moxibustion should not be performed on the right side of the chest.
- Likewise, in the spring, moxibustion should not be performed on the left side of the chest.
- Likewise, in winter, moxibustion should not be performed on the hips.
- Moxibustion is to be avoided on hot sunny days.

There also exist contraindications according to the patient's astrological sign:

- In the early afternoon for the rat
- In the late afternoon for the ox
- In the evening for the tiger
- Just before sunset for the rabbit
- On or after the sunset for the dragon, snake, horse, or sheep
- Just before dawn for the rooster or monkey
- At sunrise for the dog
- Midday (when the sun is warm) for the pig

Method

The Points for Moxibustion

The various locations on the body used for the application of heat are described in detail in Chapter 21 of the Oral Instruction Tantra. There exist two categories of points:

- Points revealed by the disorder: those points are sore or sunken when pressed. Those are suitable for moxibustion unless they are over the vulnerable points of the body.

- Points revealed by the doctor, i.e. those described in texts. There are 20 points on the back, 22 points on the front of the chest and abdomen, and 29 points on the limbs, head, and neck.

The authors feel that precise description of the moxibustion points is best conveyed through oral instruction in the appropriate clinical setting.

Type of Herb

The herb used is *spra ba (Leontopodium sp.)*. It is astringent in taste and neutral in potency. It must be harvested in the fall on an auspicious day, i.e. on the 8th, 10th, or 15th day of the lunar month. When rolled or pressed between the fingers, the herb should clump together. If it does not, it should not be used. It is not clear to the authors whether the type of mugwort used in traditional Chinese or Japanese medicine is suitable for Tibetan moxibustion.

Cone Preparation

The herb should be rolled into a small cone and applied to a smooth flat area of the skin. The size of the cone depends on the condition being treated, on the kind of patient, and on the area of the body where it is applied. The cone is lit and the doctor may blow on it to even the burning.

- For the head and trunk, the cones should be the size of the tip of the ring finger.
- For benign and malignant tumors, the cones should be the size of one half of a seed of *a ru ra* (chebulic myrobalan).
- For children, the cones should be the size of a small bean, especially if they are applied on the tip of the sternum.
- Cones applied near the spine should be no larger than the tip of the little finger.

Techniques

There exist four techniques for moxibustion:

- "Boiling": Twenty small cones are applied one after the other around a swelling or tumor.
- "Burning": Fifteen cones are applied over a given point one after the other. Each cone is placed slightly differently each time, slowly tracing a circle about the size of a pea in order to warm up a larger area. This technique is used for wind that affects the heart, phlegm, and lymph *(chu ser)*.

- "Merely applying heat": Five to seven cones are applied to one point, each cone placed slightly differently in order not to burn the skin. This is beneficial for bowel disorders, wind, urinary blockage, and cold-type infectious disorders.
- "Sudden application of heat": One very small cone is burned and removed just before leaving a scar. This technique is used with children.

Mantra Recitation

At the moment of placing the first cone, the doctor takes refuge,[22] generates bodhicitta,[23] and invokes the power of the medicine. The mantra of the Medicine Buddha[24] is then recited. This is done in order to prevent the *bla* (soul or life force) of the patient from being injured by the technique. Calendrical and astrological observances are kept for the same reason. At the end, the doctor dedicates the merit for the welfare of all sentient beings, as is customary at the end of Buddhist liturgical or contemplative practice.

Ending the Treatment

When each cone is nearly burned down, it is blown off or flicked away. After the last cone, the patient should take a few steps immediately. The patient should not drink cold water until the next morning and preferably refrain from it for a few more days, since doing so might weaken or even negate the treatment.

[22.] "Taking refuge" means reaffirming one's vows of relying on the Three Jewels, which are the Buddha, the dharma (the Buddhist doctrine), and the *sangha* (the community of lay and monastic practitioners who uphold the doctrine), to obtain lasting happiness for oneself and others.

[23.] The aspiration to be of benefit to all sentient beings without any discrimination whatsoever.

[24.] For more information on the practice of the Medicine Buddha, see Khenchen Thrangu Rinpoche 2004, cited in the bibliography.

ADDITIONAL MODALITIES

The following modalities are also described in the various chapters of the Oral Instruction Tantra that deal with the treatment of humoral and fever disorders:

Enema

Enema is used when wind affects the pelvic region and in invigoration therapy. The mild type is made of warm old butter or ghee alone. The strong type is made by adding *sgog skya* (garlic) and *rgyam tshwa* (rock salt) to the butter or ghee.

Fumigation

Fumigation is used in the treatment of wind disorders. The entire body is bathed in the steam obtained from boiling bones steeped in old wine. For this purpose a special steam-bath apparatus is necessary.

Inhalation Therapy

Inhalation therapy is used in the treatment of wind disorders. It can be performed in one of three ways: breathing the smoke of medicinal incense, breathing the vapor of medicinal herbs being boiled in water, or snuffing a finely ground medicinal powder.

Massage

Massage is used in the treatment of wind disorders and in invigoration therapy. Massage in Tibetan medicine is most often performed with fatty substances such as old sesame oil, old butter or ghee, bone marrow, the fat from marmot, etc.

Poultice

Poultices are used in the treatment of wind disorders. A medicinal herb powder is selected in accordance with the disorder being treated, then mixed with sesame oil. Lumps of the paste are placed on moxibustion points selected for the same disorder, then heat is applied.

Fomentation

Fomentation can treat wind, phlegm, and fever disorders. It entails applying cold or hot objects or compresses at specific locations on the body. Accordingly, therapies are classified into cooling and warming.

Cooling therapy can be given using *chu rdo,* a kind of round black pebble:

> A stone taken without being exposed to sun from cold water falling
> from a rock in a mountain facing north. It removes pain due to
> blood disorders (Pasang Yonten Arya 1998).

The stone *sman lcags* (magnetite) is also used in cooling fomentation. It reduces pain caused by hot conditions. Compresses with cold water or cooled-down decoctions of cooling herbs help the esophagus, eye inflammations and summertime pain and diarrhea. Cooling fomentation therapy is contraindicated for unripe fever and wind-related fever.

Warming fomentation should not be given when there is strong fever. Wind-related pain may be relieved by *dkar gong* (quartz) kept in warm Tibetan ale. Applied warm to the stomach, *so phag* (burned clay) increases digestive heat and helps manifest or ripen unripe fever, hidden fever and turbid fever.

AFTERWORD

In this proud country of the United States of America, harried and overworked people bankrupt themselves for health care[25] and still are left unsatisfied. In the name of science and professionalism, mercantilism has been allowed to run rampant. The materialistic outlook threatens to reduce all to utter powerlessness. The time has come to rediscover our human heritage of the various medical traditions, which are quite simply based on helping one another. It is only because of the perversions of modern living that we now risk losing this trove of ancient knowledge. Because real medicine is based on compassion, all medical traditions can be said to be the expression of the Medicine Buddha in his many guises. Let there be, then, enough interest on the part of patients and practitioners to keep alive this most profound system of medicine of Tibet. In this way, may people regain control of their lives and be at ease, prosperous, and free from fear.

---

25. Every thirty seconds in the United States, someone files for bankruptcy in the aftermath of a serious health problem (National Coalition on Health Care 2009; Himmelstein et al. 2005).

APPENDIXES

EXTENDED WYLIE TRANSLITERATION REFERENCE

Tibetan Alphabet

གྭ ka	ཁ kha	ག ga	ང nga
ཙ ca	ཚ cha	ཇ ja	ཉ nya
ཏ ta	ཐ tha	ད da	ན na
པ pa	ཕ pha	བ ba	མ ma
ཙ tsa	ཚ *tsha*	ཛ dza	ཝ wa
ཞ zha	ཟ za	འ 'a	ཡ ya
ར ra	ལ la	ཤ sha	ས sa
ཧ ha	ཨ a		

Extensions and Sanskrit Names

གཀྲ་ཀ་རི་	*kaNDa ka ri*
གང་གཱ་ཆུང་	*gang gA chung*
གི་ཝཾ་	*gi waM*
སྒྲོ་པུཥ་	*sgro puShpa*
ནཱ་ག་གེ་སར་	*nA ga ge sar*
པུ་ཥྐར་མཱུ་ལ་	*pu Shkara mU la*
པུཥྤ་གེ་སར་	*puShpa ge sar*
ཛཱ་ཏི་	*dzA ti*
ཡ་བཀྲ་ར་	*ya bakSha ra*
གཡའ་ཀྱི་མ་	*g.ya' kyi ma*
གཡུ་ཐོག་	*g.yu thog*
གཡེར་མ་	*g.yer ma*
ས་ རྦ་མངྒ་ལྃ་	*sarwa mangalam*
སོ་མ་རཱ་ཛ་	*so ma rA dza*
ཨིནྡྲ་	*indra*
ཨུཏྤལ་	*ut pal*

Sample Tibetan Medicine Curricula

This section is intended to give the reader examples of different approaches to the study of traditional Tibetan or *amchi* medicine. Several other curricula have been described elsewhere (Aschoff and Rösing 1997). In addition, there exist many family lineages where learning takes the form of apprenticeship from generation to generation.

The Tibetan Medical and Astrological Institute *(sman rtsis khang)*

The Tibetan Medical and Astrological Institute was founded in 1961 in McLeod Ganj, India, near Dharamsala, and started with rudimentary facilities and very little funding. It has now become a very large institution comprising fifty branch clinics in India and Nepal, research and pharmaceutical facilities, and of course a medical college.

At present the program to train Tibetan doctors lasts five years. The first four years focus mostly on theory with about four hours of class each day, and the rest of the day available for private study, optional lectures, clinical observation, helping with the preparation of pharmaceuticals, etc. Students begin to get exposed to the clinical setting in the fourth year. The fifth year comprises mostly internship with about thirty-five hours of practice per week. For extra credit, students are encouraged to memorize the First, Second, and Fourth Tantras, which they recite before their peers at the end of their training.

The Shang Shung Institute of America

Since 2005 the Shang Shung Institute in Conway, Massachusetts, has been offering the first in-depth Tibetan medicine program in North America. Its four-year program is structured as follows (Tibetan Medicine Program 2007):

Core foundation studies, covering the Four Tantras	1,540 hours
Tibetan language and culture	448 hours
Clinical practicum	252 hours
Optional six-month internship at the Northeast Traditional Tibetan Hospital in Qinghai, China	320 hours

The British Association of Traditional Tibetan Medicine

The British Association of Traditional Tibetan Medicine is a branch of the European Herbal and Traditional Medicine Practitioners Association, which developed the following curricular recommendation for accrediting all herbal practitioners. Their standards include specific requirements for Tibetan medicine but share a common format with the other herbal systems they oversee (European Herbal Association 2007):

Human Sciences	250 hours
Nutrition	80 hours
Clinical Sciences	350 hours
Plant Chemistry and Pharmacology	80 hours
Pharmacognosy and Dispensing	100 hours
Practitioner Development and Ethics	150 hours
Practitioner Research	150 hours
The specific herbal tradition	1,150 hours
Clinical Practice	500 hours

BIBLIOGRAPHY

Tibetan Medicine

Aschoff, Jürgen, and Ina Rösing, eds. 1997. *Tibetan medicine: East meets west, west meets east.* Ulm, Germany: Fabri Verlag

Clark, Barry. 1995. *The Quintessence Tantras of Tibetan medicine.* Ithaca, NY: Snow Lion.

Dash, Vaidya Bhagwan. 2001. *Encyclopaedia of Tibetan medicine (7 vols.).* Delhi: Sri Satguru.

Lobsang Rapgay. 1985. A guide to Tibetan medical urinalysis. In *Tibetan medicine.* Dharamsala, India: Library of Tibetan Works and Archives; reprinted in *Acupuncture and Electro-therapeutics Research* 11 (1986): 25–43.

Men Tsee Khang. 1997. *Fundamentals of Tibetan medicine.* Dharamsala, India: Men Tsee Khang. ISBN 81-86419-04-7.

Parfionovitch, Yuri, Fernand Meyer, and Gyurme Dorje, eds. 1992. *Tibetan medical paintings.* London: Serindia.

Shang Shung Institute. 2007. *Tibetan medicine program academic catalog (draft).* Conway, MA: Shang Shung Institute.

Tenzing (sic) Dakpa. 2007. *Science of healing: A comprehensive commentary on the Root Tantra and diagnostic techniques of Tibetan medicine.* Pittsburgh: Dorrance.

Thubten Phuntsog. 2001. *Three-year Tibetan medicine course transcript (draft).* Conway, MA: Shang Shung Institute.

Yeshi Donden. 1986. *Health through balance.* Ithaca, NY: Snow Lion.

Zhen Yang and Cai Jingfeng. 2005. *China's Tibetan medicine.* Beijing: Foreign Languages Press. ISBN 7-119-3350-6.

Tibetan Herbs and Foods

Clark, Barry. 2000. *Problems of identifying and translating materia medica used in Tibetan medicine.* Kalimpong, India: AyurVijnana VII.

Dawa, A. 1999. *Clear mirror of Tibetan medicinal plants.* Rome: Tibet Domani.

Joshi, Kamal K., and Sanu Devi Joshi. 2006. *Medicinal and aromatic plants used in Nepal, Tibet and trans-Himalayan region.* Bloomington, IL: AuthorHouse.

Kletter, Christa, and Monika Kriechbaum. 2001. *Tibetan medicinal plants.* Stuttgart: Medpharm.

Men-Tsee-Khang. 2006. *Tibetan medical dietary book: Vol. I.* Dharamsala, India: Tibetan Medical and Astrological Institute. ISBN 81-86419-54-3.

Molvray, Mia. 1988. A glossary of Tibetan medicinal plants. In *Tibetan medicine.* Dharamsala, India: Library of Tibetan Works and Archives.

Pasang Yonten Arya. 1998. *Dictionary of Tibetan materia medica.* Delhi: Motilal Banarsidass.

Tendzin Dakpa. 2007. *Tibetan medicinal plants.* New Delhi: Paljor. ISBN 81-86230-56-4.

Tsewang Tsarong. 1994. *Tibetan medicinal plants.* Kalimpong, India: Tibetan Medical Publications.

Tibetan Herbal Formulas

Dash, Vaidya Bhagwan. 1994. *Pharmacopoeia of Tibetan medicine.* Delhi: Sri Satguru.

Dawa, A. 2009. *Clear mirror of Tibetan medicinal plants, vol. II.* Dharamsala, India: Tibetan Medical and Astrological Institute. ISBN 81-86419-61-6.

Men-Tsee-Khang. 1995. *Guide to the exhibition on Tibetan medicine and astrology.* Dharamsala, India. ISBN 81-86419-03-9.

Smanla T. Phuntsog. 2006. *Ancient metria* (sic) *medica.* New Delhi: Paljor.

Tsewang Tsarong. 1986. *Handbook of traditional Tibetan drugs.* Kalimpong, India: Tibetan Medical Publications.

Chinese Herbs

中华本草，藏药卷 (*Chinese materia medica, Tibetan medicine volume;* in Chinese). 2002. 上海科学技出版社 (Shanghai: Shanghai Scientific and Technical Publishing). ISBN 7-5323-6628-6.

Bensky, Dan, and Andrew Gamble. 1986. *Chinese herbal medicine: Materia medica.* Seattle: Eastland.

Chang Hson-Mou and Paul Pui-Hay But. 1986–1987. *Pharmacology and applications of Chinese materia medica (2 volumes).* Singapore: World Scientific.

Ayurvedic Herbs

Caldecott, Todd. 2006. *Ayurveda: The divine science of life.* Philadelphia: Elsevier.

Kareem, Abdul. 1997. *Plants in Ayurveda (A compendium of botanical and Sanskrit names).* Bangalore: Foundation for the Revitalisation of Local Health Traditions.

Tirtha, Swami Sada Shiva. 1998. *The Ayurveda encyclopedia.* Bayville, NY: Ayurveda Holistic Center.

Williamson, Elizabeth. 2002. *Major herbs of Ayurveda.* London: Churchill Livingstone.

Other Herbal Reference Sources

Badola, Hemant K., and Mohinder Pal. 2002. Endangered medicinal plant species in Himachal Pradesh. *Current Science* 83 (7): 797–8.

European Herbal and Traditional Medicine Practitioners Association. 2007. *The Core curriculum for herbal and traditional medicine.* Tewkesbury, UK.

Gruenwald, Joerg, Thomas Bendler, and Christof Jaenicke, eds. 2000. *PDR for herbal medicines.* Montvale, NJ: Medical Economics Co.

IUCN. 2009. The IUCN red list of threatened species. http://www.iucnredlist.org/.

Ross, Ivan A. 1999, 2001, 2005. *Medicinal plants of the world (3 volumes).* Totowa, NJ: Humana.

Willard, Terry. 1991. *The wild rose scientific herbal.* Calgary: Wild Rose College of Natural Healing.

World Health Organization. 2007. *WHO monographs on selected medicinal plants, volume 3.* Geneva: WHO.

Buddhism

Chögyam Trungpa. 1993. *Training the Mind.* Boston: Shambhala.

Khenchen Thrangu Rinpoche. 2004. *Medicine Buddha Teachings.* Ithaca, NY: Snow Lion.

Liberating animals (internal publication). 2005. Portland, OR: Foundation for the Preservation of the Mahayana Tradition.

Walshe, Maurice, trans. 1987. *The long discourses of the Buddha.* Somerville, MA: Wisdom.

Miscellaneous References

Garson, Nathaniel, and David Germano. 2004. Extended Wylie transliteration scheme. Tibetan and Himalayan Digital Library. http://www.thdl.org/.

Heineman, Paul G. 1921. *Milk.* London: W. B. Saunders.

Himmelstein, D. U., E. Warren, D. Thorne, and S. Woolhandler. Illness and injury as contributors to bankruptcy. *Health Affairs* February 2, 2005.

The Merck index, tenth edition. 1983. Rahway, NJ: Merck & Co.

National Coalition on Health Care. 2009. Health insurance costs. http://www.nchc.org/.

Tournadre, Nicolas. 2003. *Manual of standard Tibetan.* Ithaca, NY: Snow Lion.

Books in Tibetan

། །བདུད་རྩི་སྙིང་པོ་ཡན་ལག་བརྒྱད་པ་གསང་བ་མན་ངག་གི་རྒྱུད་ཅེས་བྱ་བ་བཞུགས་སོ།།
མཚོ་སྔོན་མི་རིགས་པར་འདེབས་བཟོ་གྲྭ་ནས་པར་བཏབ།

(The Four Tantras, *mtsho sngon,* 1982 edition)

། །གསོ་བ་རིག་པའི་བསྟན་བཅོས་སྨན་བླའི་དགོངས་རྒྱན་རྒྱུད་བཞིའི་གསལ་བྱེད་བཻ་ཌཱུར་སྔོན་པོའི་མལ་ལི་ཀ་ཞེས་བྱ་བ་
བཞུགས་སོ།།

(The Blue Beryl commentary on the Four Tantras)

། །ཁོག་འབུགས་འགྱེལ་པ་འབུམ་ནག་གསལ་སྒྲོན། ཌོ་ན་ཌ་རིས་བཙལས།།

(Commentary on the Second Tantra by *sum spon ye shes*)

། །གསོ་བ་རིག་པའི་ཚིག་མཛོད་ག.ཡུ་ཐོག་དགོངས་རྒྱན།།

(Medical dictionary by *g.yu thog*)

། །གཉིས་བསྒྱུར་འཆི་མེད་ནོར་བུའི་ཕྲེང་བ (མ་ཡིག) དང་ མན་ངག་སྙིང་གི་ནོར་བུ (བུ་ཡིག) བཞུགས་སོ།།

(Classic formulary by *karma nges don bstan 'dzin 'phrin las rab rgyas*)

། །སྨན་སྦྱོར་གྱི་ནུས་པ་ཕྱོགས་བསྡུས་ཕན་བདེའི་ལེགས་བཤད་ཅེས་བྱ་བ་བཞུགས་སོ།།

(Formulary published by *sman rtsi khang,* 1995)

INDEXES

Herb Index by Tibetan Drug Name

HERB INDEX BY LATIN NAME

*Page numbers in **boldface** indicate monographs.*

HERB INDEX BY ENGLISH DRUG NAME

*Page numbers in **boldface** indicate monographs.*

Formula Index by Tibetan Name

Formula Index by English Name

General Index